LABORATORY

MAJOR PROBLEMS IN INTERNAL MEDICINE

Published

Cline: Cancer Chemotherapy (*Second Edition*), by Cline and Haskell,
  now available separately from the publisher
Shearn: Sjögren's Syndrome
Cogan: Ophthalmic Manifestations of Systemic Vascular Disease
Williams: Rheumatoid Arthritis as a Systemic Disease
Cluff, Caranasos and Stewart: Clinical Problems with Drugs
Fries and Holman: Systemic Lupus Erythematosus
Kass: Pernicious Anemia

In Preparation

Bray: The Obese Patient
Gorlin: Coronary Artery Disease
Ingbar: Pathophysiology and Diagnosis of Disorders of the Thyroid
Krugman and Ward: Viral Hepatitis
Potts: Disorders of Calcium Metabolism
Felig: Diabetes Mellitus
Bunn, Forget and Ranney: Normal and Abnormal Hemoglobins
Sleisenger and Brandborg: Malabsorption
Havel and Kane: Diagnosis and Treatment of Hyperlipidemias
Siltzbach: Sarcoidosis
Scheinberg and Sternlieb: Wilson's Disease and Copper Metabolism
Atkins and Bodel: Fever
Lieber and De Carli: Medical Aspects of Alcoholism
Merrill: Glomerulonephritis
Goldberg: The Scientific Basis and Practical Use of Diuretics
Laragh: Reversible Hypertension
Kilbourne: Influenza
Deykin: Diseases of the Platelets
Schwartz and Lergier: Immunosuppressive Therapy
Cohen: Amyloidosis
Seegmiller: Gout
Weinstein: Infective Endocarditis
Sasahara: Pulmonary Embolism
Zieve and Levin: Disorders of Hemostasis
Salmon: Multiple Myeloma

ABRAHAM I. BRAUDE, M.D., Ph.D.

Professor of Medicine and Pathology, Chief Division
of Infectious Diseases, University of California, San Diego;
Director of Microbiology, University Hospital

ANTIMICROBIAL DRUG THERAPY

VOLUME

VIII

IN THE SERIES

MAJOR PROBLEMS IN INTERNAL MEDICINE

Lloyd H. Smith, Jr., M.D., *Editor*

W. B. SAUNDERS COMPANY • PHILADELPHIA • LONDON • TORONTO • 1976

W. B. Saunders Company: West Washington Square
Philadelphia, PA   19105

12 Dyott Street
London, WC1A 1DB

833 Oxford Street
Toronto, Ontario M8Z 5T9, Canada

Library of Congress Cataloging in Publication Data

Braude, Abraham I.

Antimicrobial Drug Therapy

(Major problems in internal medicine; v. 8)

Includes index.

1. Anti-infective agents.   I.   Title.   [DNLM: 1. Anti-infective agents—Therapeutic use. W1 MA492T v. 8 / QV250 B825a]

RM262.B7   615'.58   75-19842
ISBN 0-7216-1918-5

Antimicrobial Drug Therapy   ISBN   0-7216-1918-5

Last digit is the print number: 9   8   7   6   5   4   3   2   1

FOREWORD

We are surrounded by microorganisms for weal or woe. Fortunately most of them do us no harm and at best work prodigiously and silently on our behalf. When bacteria or viruses do invade they generally come off second best against a versatile defense of antibodies and phagocytes. Nevertheless, the infectious diseases are still the most common of man's afflictions. In a national health survey almost 50,000,000 cases of acute infectious or parasitic diseases were reported in the United States in 1969. Since our current armamentarium is firmly based on the principles of bacteriology and immunology which were established long before antimicrobial agents were discovered or developed, it can be said that the conquest of the infectious diseases, incomplete though it is, marks the greatest therapeutic triumph of the biomedical sciences in the past century.

Several years ago it was estimated that over 22,000 drug products were being marketed. The number seems unlikely to diminish. Antibiotics account for approximately 15 per cent of prescriptions filled in the United States annually.[3] Virtually all physicians in the practice of medicine or any of its specialties are called upon to treat infectious diseases with these agents. How well is this responsibility being discharged? Most evidence would suggest that physicians have great difficulty in keeping up with the confusing array of antimicrobial agents and their proper use in therapy. Not only are there many new agents, but the target may be a moving one, as microorganisms develop their own adaptations for survival in the form of resistance to our "magic bullets," as Ehrlich termed chemotherapeutic agents. Drugs interact in a variety of occult ways to reinforce or to neutralize. They have many direct and indirect adverse reactions, as summarized here for antibiotics and as detailed in another monograph in this series.[1] Surveys have shown that as a result of these and other variables large numbers of physicians fail to use antibiotics properly. One such survey has recently received wide publicity in the national press.[2]

In this monograph, *Antimicrobial Drug Therapy*, Dr. Abraham I. Braude has presented a succinct summary of the scientific basis for the clinical use of these agents. The premise on which the book is based has been stated in his introductory remarks, "I feel there is still a need for a basic understanding of the chemistry, mode of action, spectrum, pharmacology, and toxicity of the many antimicrobial drugs if they are to be used to the best advantage in clinical practice." Dr. Braude is eminently well qualified for this undertaking from the perspective of one who has had a distinguished career in the disciplines of infectious diseases and microbiology. Within these seven chapters Dr. Braude presents a lucid and rational guide to the antibiotics and their use in medicine. *Antimicrobial Drug Therapy* should therefore be of value to virtually everyone in medical practice.

LLOYD H. SMITH, JR., M.D.

REFERENCES

1. Cluff LE, Caranasos GJ, Stewart RB: *Clinical Problems with Drugs.* Philadelphia, W.B. Saunders Co., 1975.
2. Neu HC, Howrey SP: Testing the physician's knowledge of antibiotic use. N Engl J Med 293:1291–1295, 1975.
3. Stolley PD, Becker MH, McEvilla JD, et al: Drug prescribing and use in an American community. Ann Intern Med 76:537–540, 1972.

PREFACE

The idea behind this book is that a doctor practices better medicine if he understands the scientific basis of what he is doing. For this reason I have tried to present a set of premises leading to the logical use of drugs in the treatment of infection.

My chief premise is the germ theory of disease: that specific infections are caused by specific microbes and that a drug is best selected for its ability to destroy them. Simple as this approach may seem, it is not in keeping with the practice of many physicians who use drugs to treat clinical entities without regard for the specific cause. I am often asked for the best treatment of pneumonia, diarrhea, meningitis, or cystitis, instead of pneumococcal, *Shigella*, meningococcal, or *Escherichia coli* infections. I am even asked about the best all-purpose remedy for everything—the best "broad-spectrum" antibiotic or drug combination to be used for obscure fever or infections, or for prevention of any and all postoperative complications. The time may come when such a panacea is available. The spectra of the penicillins are becoming so wide, now that such organisms as *Pseudomonas* are susceptible to carbenicillin, that one of these drugs may one day become the cure for all infections. At the time of this writing the full therapeutic potential of a trimethoprim-sulfonamide combination is being explored, and I am amazed at its activity and clinical value for disorders caused by organisms ranging from bacteria to protozoa. But so far no single treatment for every infection, or nearly every infection, has been discovered, and I feel there is still a need for a basic understanding of the chemistry, mode of action, spectrum, pharmacology, and toxicity of many antimicrobial drugs if they are to be used to the best advantage in clinical practice.

In putting this information together, I soon realized how much we owe some of our contemporary clinical investigators for asking and answering important questions about many of these drugs. Wesley Spink was a pioneer in working out the usefulness of sulfonamides and in exploring the problem of penicillin resistance to staphylococcal infections. Charles Rammelkamp did much to establish a proper understanding of the treatment of streptococcal infections. William Kirby not only discovered staphylococcal

penicillinase and developed with Bauer the standard disk method for
testing antibiotic sensitivities, but also worked out the pharmacology of
many antibiotics. Maxwell Finland and his associates have compiled a
prodigious collection of invaluable data on microbial drug susceptibility,
and much of the information in this book dealing with antibiotic sensitivity
is derived from their work. Calvin Kunin is largely responsible for our
concepts of antibiotic therapy in renal failure and antibiotic binding by
proteins and tissues.

Our debt is even greater to the biochemists, microbiologists, and
molecular biologists who created the groundwork for chemotherapy. In
their discovery of penicillin and the sulfonamides, Fleming and Domagh so
overshadowed their successors that we tend to overlook the brilliant contributions of later investigators who expanded the early findings. Florey
and his colleagues at Oxford discovered how to isolate penicillin in a relatively pure state (after Fleming gave up because of its instability) and went
on to demonstrate its value in treating human infections. More recently
Batchelor set the stage for the semisynthetic penicillins by isolating
6-aminopenicillanic acid from the fermentation medium, and Robinson
described methicillin, the first significant penicillin with resistance to
staphylococcal penicillinase. The mode of action of penicillin and the nature
of its selective toxicity have been greatly clarified by the work of Leder-
berg, Park, and Strominger. The importance of resistance transfer among
gram-negative bacteria and its role in epidemic drug resistance were first
worked out by the Japanese scientists Akiba, Mitsuhaski, and Watanabe.
And for drugs active against protozoa and worms, I found the extensive
work of Ernest Bueding an infallible source of basic information.

I have discussed many other contributions to the field of antimicrobial
drug therapy that relieve suffering from infection. If nothing else, I hope
this book will make the practicing physician more aware of the ideas
responsible for the success doctors enjoy in treating infections with drugs.

ABRAHAM I. BRAUDE

CONTENTS

CHAPTER 1

DESCRIPTION OF ANTIMICROBIAL DRUGS

Antimicrobial drugs may no longer be classified according to the organisms they inhibit because their spectra can be broadened by minor adjustments in structure or dosage. Classification of antibiotics and synthetic antimicrobial drugs is based instead on chemical structure or biochemical effects. Since the biochemical effects are considered in the next chapter, "Mechanisms of Action," a chemical classification will be presented here. All antimicrobial drugs are ring compounds; otherwise, the various groups have little structural similarity.

THE PEPTIDES

The penicillins, cephalosporins, bacitracin, and polymyxins are the most important peptide antibiotics. Their molecular weight seldom exceeds 3000. For this reason they are too small to be antigenic and stimulate neutralizing antibodies that would cause them to lose activity with continued administration. Small nonantigenic peptide antibiotics are a lucky evolutionary by-product in the molds and bacteria that produce these antimicrobial agents. They are small because they are synthesized by a pathway that does not depend on the elaborate system for coding amino acids and their sequences required for protein synthesis. It is likely that microbial peptides, including peptide antibiotics, evolved before the process of protein synthesis via nucleic-acid coding on ribosomes. Since the functions performed by peptides were later taken over by microbial proteins, the peptides can be regarded as "fossils."[1] The fact that the majority of these antibiotics have a cyclic structure is also consistent with the idea that they once performed a functional role in microbial metabolism because cyclic structures are found in enzymes and other functional proteins.

1

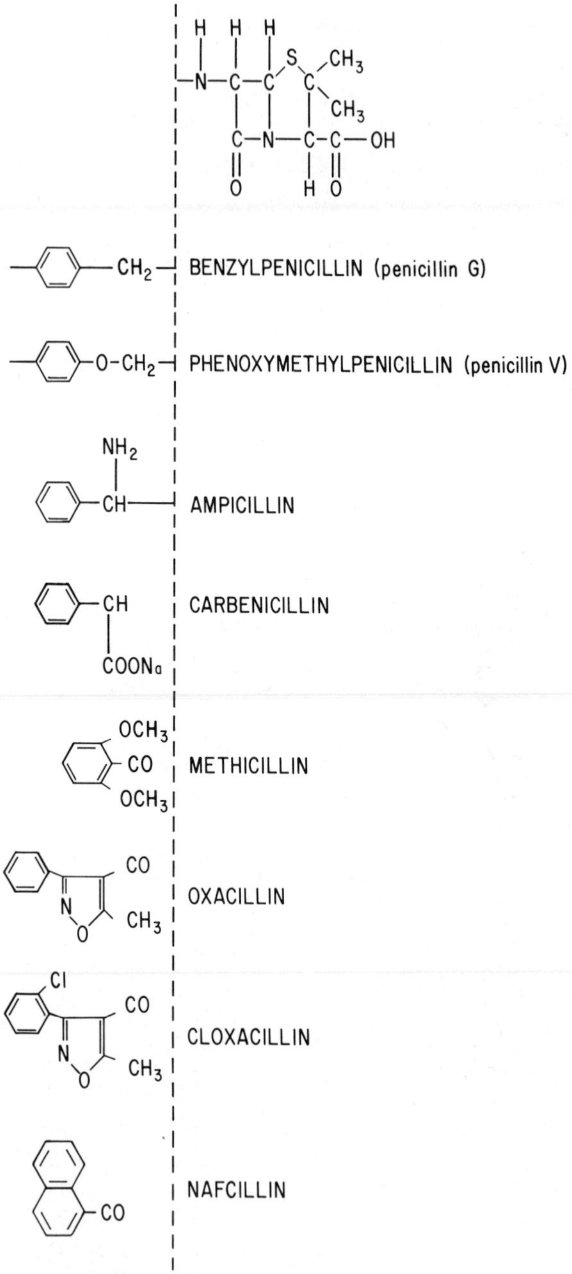

Figure 1–1. The side chains responsible for the biologic differences in each of the penicillins are shown to the left of the dotted line, and 6-aminopenicillanic acid is on the right. The last four side chains protect the β-lactam ring from the action of penicillinase.

The Penicillins

The common nucleus of the penicillins is 6-aminopenicillanic acid, a cyclic dipeptide of L-cysteine and D-valine (Fig. 1–1). These are arranged in a basic structure consisting of a thiazolidine ring joined to a β-lactam ring. Individual penicillins differ with respect to the side chains attached to the common nucleus. The most important of the naturally occurring penicillins is penicillin G, containing a benzyl side chain (Fig. 1–1). Penicillin V is obtained when phenoxyacetic acid is added as a precursor to the fermentation medium so that a phenoxymethyl side chain becomes attached to the penicillin nucleus. This compound is well suited for oral use because of its resistance to gastric acid. Other penicillins are prepared by the synthetic addition of various groups as side chains to 6-aminopenicillanic acid after it has been isolated from *Penicillium* fermentation media. Depending on their chemical structure, these side chains can broaden the antimicrobial spectrum, protect the penicillin nucleus from acid hydrolysis, or protect it against penicillinase. In ampicillin, for example, the presence of an amino group in the phenyl radical of benzylpenicillin produces a compound both resistant to acid and more active against gram-negative bacteria than penicillin G. If a carboxyl group is introduced instead, as in carbenicillin, the spectrum is altered so that the compound becomes the only penicillin derivative with activity against *Pseudomonas aeruginosa*. None of these modifications, however, confers resistance to staphylococcal penicillinase. This was first accomplished in the synthesis of methicillin by the introduction of methoxy groups at positions 2 and 6 on the benzyl ring so that affinity of the substrate site for penicillinase is reduced 10,000 times.[11] This modification did not achieve acid resistance, but the synthesis of isoxazolyl penicillin introduced a series of products with combined resistance to penicillinase and gastric acid. Oxacillin and dicloxacillin are the most widely used of these doubly resistant penicillins. The structural modifications of semisynthetic penicillins are illustrated in Figure 1–1.

The Cephalosporins

The common nucleus of the cephalosporins resembles 6-aminopenicillanic acid but differs by having a dihydrothiazine ring, instead of a thiazolidine ring, attached to the β-lactam ring (Fig. 1–2). The active nucleus, known as 7-aminocephalosporanic acid, can also be manipulated chemically to yield more active and useful derivatives.[6] The basic advantages of the cephalosporin nucleus are its innate resistance to staphylococcal penicillinase and its safety in patients with allergy to penicillin. These properties are retained in cephalothin (Fig. 1–3), in which the side chain at the 7-position increases its potency and range of activity. Another derivative, cephalexin (Fig. 1–3), has a different side chain at the 7-position that confers resistance to gastric acid and allows good absorption from the alimentary tract. Cefazolin (Fig. 1–3), with substitutions at both the 7- and 3-positions, can be injected intramuscularly without pain and possesses greater activity than cephalothin against certain bacteria.

4 DESCRIPTION OF ANTIMICROBIAL DRUGS

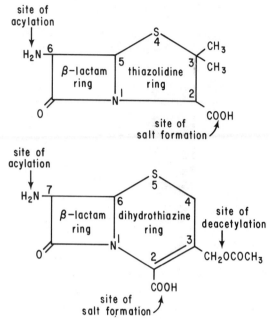

Figure 1–2. Comparison of penicillin nucleus, 6-aminopenicillanic acid (upper figure), with cephalosporin nucleus, 7-aminocephalosporanic acid (lower diagram). The main difference in the two compounds is the thiazolidine ring in penicillin and the dihydrothiazine ring in the cephalosporins. Most penicillin derivatives are produced by addition of side chains at the acylation site. Cephalosporin derivatives vary in the chemical groups at the acylation site, and at the deacetylation site as well.

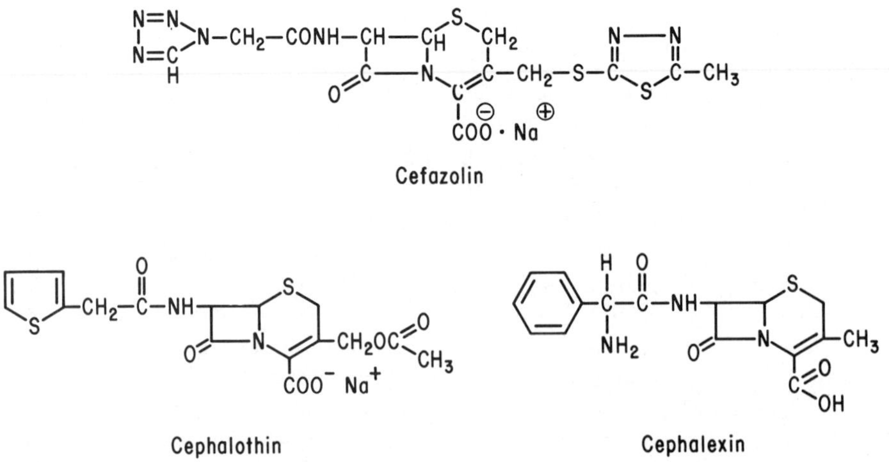

Cefazolin

Cephalothin

Cephalexin

Figure 1–3. Structural formulas of three important cephalosporin derivatives illustrate differences in side chains at acylation and deacetylation sites.

BACITRACIN A

Figure 1–4. Like penicillin, bacitracin A contains a thiazolidine ring. It is a condensation product of isoleucine and cysteine, in contrast to that of penicillin which contains D-valine and L-cysteine. Bacitracin lacks the β-lactam ring of penicillin.

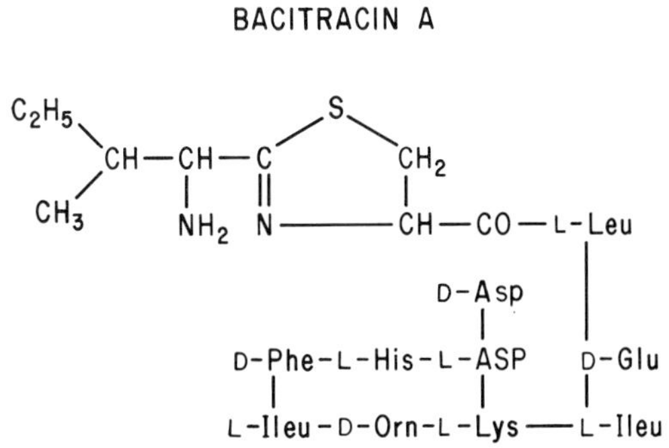

$$
\begin{array}{c}
C_2H_5 \\
\backslash \\
CH-CH-C \\
/ \quad | \quad \| \\
CH_3 \quad NH_2 \quad N
\end{array}
\begin{array}{c}
S \\
\diagup \quad \diagdown \\
\quad\quad CH_2 \\
\quad\quad | \\
CH-CO-\text{L-Leu}
\end{array}
$$

D-Asp

D-Phe–L-His–L-ASP   D-Glu

L-Ileu–D-Orn–L-Lys——L-Ileu

Bacitracin

This antibiotic is produced by a strain of *Bacillus subtilis,* which was isolated from the dirty compound fracture of a girl named Tracy and called "bacitracin" out of joint deference to the bacillus and patient.[8] The antibiotic consists of a mixture of polypeptides, the most important of which is bacitracin A. Like the penicillins, it contains a thiazolidine ring but does not have their β-lactam ring. In bacitracin A the thiazolidine ring is a condensation product of isoleucine and a cysteine residue and is attached through L-leucine to a peptide composed of D- and L-amino acids (Fig. 1–4).

POLYMYXIN B

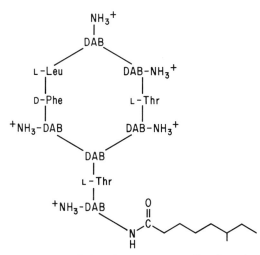

Figure 1–5. Diaminobutyric acid (DAB) is present in all polymyxins, including colistin (polymyxin E). The terminal residue of DAB is acetylated by 6-methyloctanoic acid, the C9 fatty acid at the bottom of the structural formula. The cationic α-amino group of DAB and the hydrophobic fatty acid are responsible for the surface-active properties of the cationic detergent.

The Polymyxins

These cyclic polypeptides are also produced by a spore-forming aerobic bacillus, *Bacillus polymyxa*. Their detergent activity on bacteria can be attributed to two unique components: an amino acid, α,γ-diaminobutyric acid (DAB), and a C9 fatty acid, 6-methyloctanoic acid (Fig. 1–5). The cationic α-amino groups of DAB and the hydrophobic side chain of the fatty acid give the polymyxins the surface-active properties of a cationic detergent. Only two of the polymyxins, B and E, are used in clinical medicine. Polymyxin E is generally known as colistin.

THE AMINOGLYCOSIDES

The aminoglycosides are derived from different species of *Streptomyces* and are composed of amino sugars. In contrast to penicillin, they are organic bases rather than acids. Streptomycin, neomycin, kanamycin, and paromomycin—listed in order of discovery—are all members of this group. They resemble each other because of the inositol residue and the prominent basic groups, ranging from three in streptomycin to six in neomycin. They differ in the sugars attached to inositol and in the guanidine groups of streptomycin (Fig. 1–6). This similarity in structure accounts for common toxic effects on patients and bacteria.

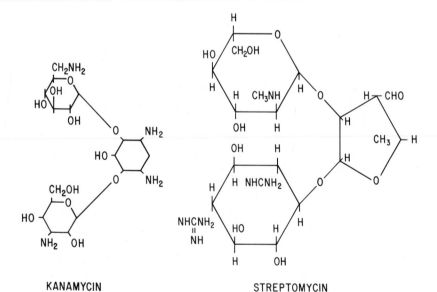

KANAMYCIN   STREPTOMYCIN

Figure 1–6. The basic structure of the aminoglycosides, illustrated by kanamycin and streptomycin, is that of a polycationic compound composed of amino sugars and connected by glycosidic linkages. In streptomycin, the inositol residue common to both compounds is in the form of streptidine (the bottom sugar with two guanido groups) and in kanamycin it is deoxystreptamine (the central sugar with amino groups).

Gentamicin is structurally similar to these aminoglycosides but is produced by a species of *Micromonospora* rather than *Streptomyces*. It has an inositol residue with two amino sugars and is a complex of three antibiotics (designated C_1, C_2, and C_{1A}) which differ in structure only by one or two methyl groups.

THE TETRACYCLINES

The tetracyclines are so named because their common hydro-naphthacene nucleus contains four fused rings (Fig. 1–7). Chlortetracycline (Aureomycin) was the first tetracycline compound described, and oxytetracycline (Terramycin) was discovered two years later in 1950. Both compounds were produced by strains of *Streptomyces*. Although tetracycline was made by the catalytic reduction of chlortetracycline, all other compounds in this group are named in relation to the basic structure of tetracycline. In chlortetracycline a hydrogen is replaced by chlorine, and in oxytetracycline it is replaced by a hydroxyl ion. Demeclocycline (Declomycin) is chlortetracycline without the 6-methyl group, and doxycycline is oxytetracycline without the 6-hydroxyl group. These minor structural differences have less effect on their antimicrobial spectra than on stability in solution and pharmacologic properties. Chlortetracycline not only is less stable than the other tetracyclines but is the least stable of any important antibiotic.

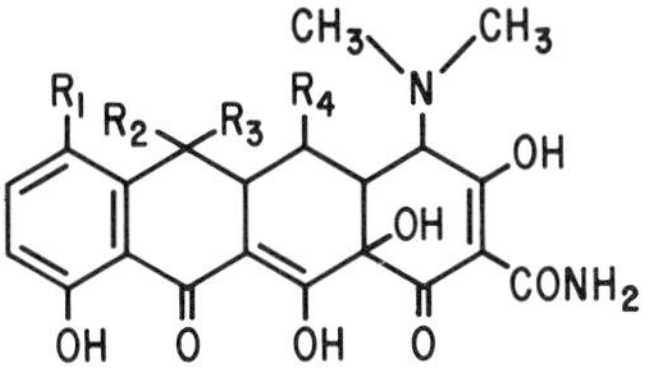

	R_1	R_2	R_3	R_4
Tetracycline	H	CH_3	OH	H
Oxytetracycline	H	CH_3	OH	OH
Doxycycline	H	CH_3	H	OH
Methacycline	H	CH_2		OH
Chlortetracycline	Cl	CH_3	OH	H
Demethylchlor-tetracycline	Cl	H	OH	H
Minocycline	$N(CH_3)_2$	H	H	H

Figure 1–7. The compounds in this group are named in relation to the basic structure of tetracycline and on the basis of substituted chemical groups at one or more of the four R positions.

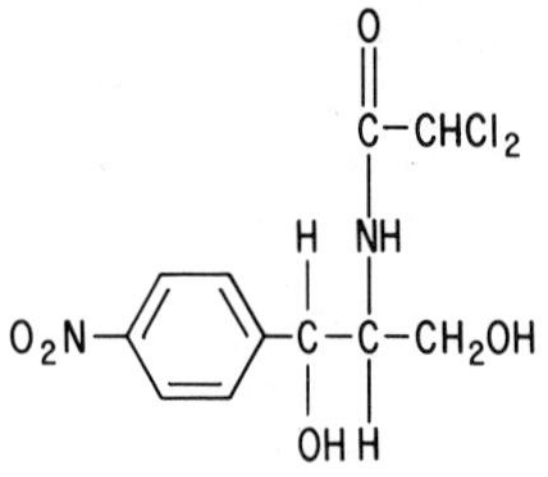

Figure 1–8. Chloramphenicol is the only naturally occurring antibiotic with nitrobenzene in its structure, a property that may account for its tendency to cause aplastic anemia.

CHLORAMPHENICOL

CHLORAMPHENICOL

Chloramphenicol is the only naturally occurring antibiotic with nitrobenzene in its structure (Fig. 1–8). This chemical grouping probably accounts for its toxicity to both bacteria and patients. Its tendency to cause aplastic anemia is explained by its benzene ring, a component of most organic substances involved in that disorder. Its ability to compete with messenger RNA for ribosomal binding is explained by its spatial similarity to uridine-5-phosphate.

THE MACROLIDES

Erythromycin, isolated from *Streptomyces erythreus*, is the only important member of the macrolides. The basic structure is a large lactone ring to which unusual sugars are attached (Fig. 1–9). The term "macrolide" refers to the large ring, formed from a chain of 14 to 20 carbon atoms by lactone condensation of a carboxyl and hydroxyl group. The other 37 macrolides, such as oleandomycin, spiramycin, kitasamycin, and carbomycin, differ from erythromycin both in the structure of the lactone ring and in the attached sugars. Since the other macrolides have the same spectrum but are less potent than erythromycin, they are not widely used.

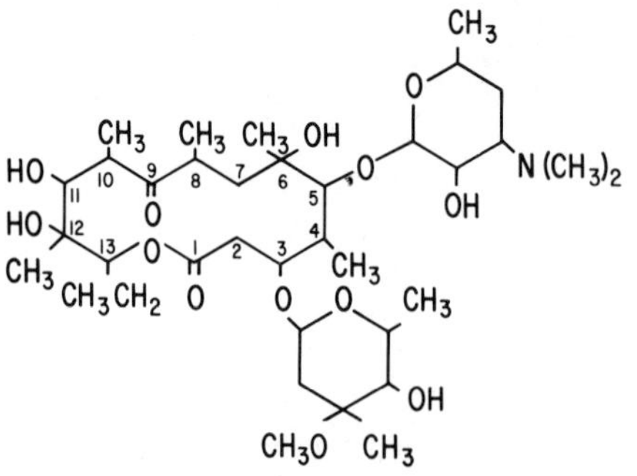

Figure 1–9. Erythromycin is the only important member of a group of 37 different compounds known as macrolides. The term "macrolide" refers to the large lactone ring formed from a chain of 14 to 20 carbon atoms by lactone condensation.

ERYTHROMYCIN

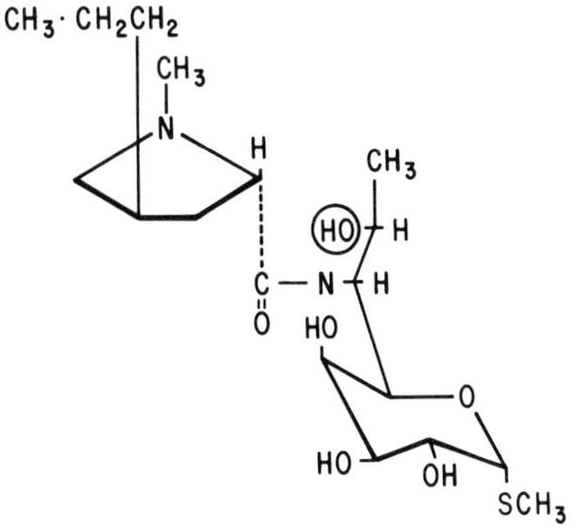

$$CH_3 \cdot CH_2CH_2$$

LINCOMYCIN

Figure 1–10. The sulfur-containing amino acid, methyl-α-thiol lincosaminide, is named for the parent compound which was obtained from a mold growing in Lincoln, Nebraska. Note total dissimilarity of lincomycin from macrolides (Fig. 1–9). The circle indicates the 7-hydroxyl group where a chloro group is substituted in clindamycin.

LINCOMYCIN

Despite striking similarity in the biologic effects of lincomycin and erythromycin, their chemical structures are totally dissimilar. In contrast to the macrolides, lincomycin consists of an amino acid joined to a sulfur-containing amino sugar. The amino acid is trans-L-4-*n*-propyl hygric acid, and the amino sugar is methyl-α-thiol lincosaminide (Fig. 1–10).

Clindamycin is a synthetic modification of lincomycin. As indicated by its chemical name, 7-chloro-7-deoxylincomycin, clindamycin is produced by a 7-chloro substitution of the 7(R)-hydroxyl group of the parent compound, lincomycin. These modifications in structure appear to increase absorption, blood levels, and antibacterial activity.

THE RIFAMYCINS

The rifamycin antibiotics are fermentation products of *Streptomyces mediterranei*. Their basic structure is an aromatic ring compound spanned by an aliphatic bridge. The most active of the original compounds, rifamycin B, was not well absorbed after ingestion. After the chemical structure of various rifamycins was determined in 1963, it was possible to synthesize a great many semisynthetic derivatives.[13] At the time of this writing, rifampin is the most important of these because it is orally effective in tuberculosis and leprosy, and in infections by various gram-negative and gram-positive bacteria. The special features of rifampin, shown in Figure 1–11, are the double ring compound, the long aliphatic bridge, and the side chain: $CH = N - N \quad N - CH_3$. The ring is a naphthohydroquinone and is the chemical grouping responsible for the red color of the antibiotic. The importance of the rifamycins lies not only in their currently important derivative, rifampin, but also in the great potential for new derivatives with activity against many different microorganisms, including viruses and fungi.

RIFAMPIN

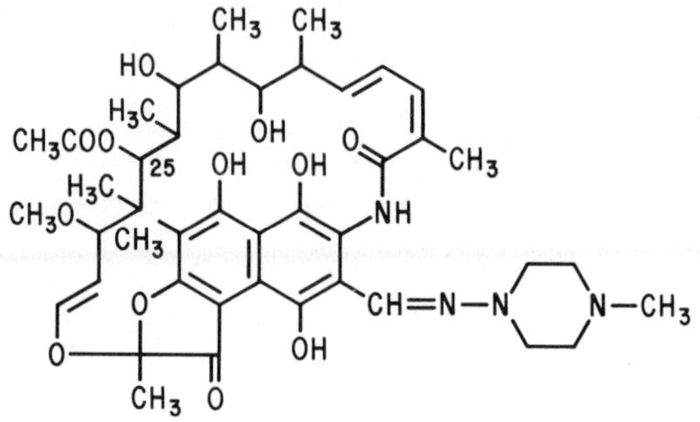

Figure 1–11. The basic structure of rifampin is the double ring compound spanned by a long aliphatic bridge, and the side chain.

VANCOMYCIN

Among antibiotics of clinical value, vancomycin is the only one of unknown structure. It is a large molecule with a molecular weight in the range of 3500 and contains sugars and amino acids of indeterminate structure.

GRISEOFULVIN

Although derived from *Penicillium* molds, griseofulvin is active against fungi rather than bacteria. Discovered in 1939 in London, griseofulvin was used against plant fungi before its value against human dermatophytes was demonstrated.[12] It has a spirocyclic structure formed from acetate units (Fig. 1–12).

THE POLYENES

Amphotericin B and nystatin are the two important members of the polyenes. These antibiotics are classified as polyenes because the molecules contain a series of carbon atoms with four or five conjugated double bonds. Nystatin and amphotericin also possess the aminodeoxyhexose, mycosa-

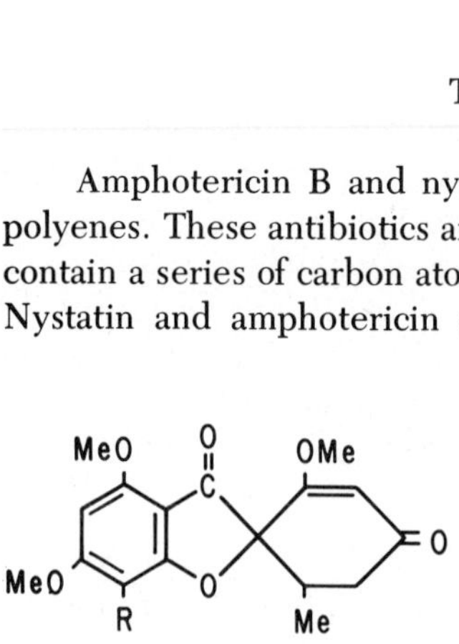

Figure 1–12. Griseofulvin is a spirocyclic compound formed from acetate units.

GRISEOFULVIN

PARTIAL STRUCTURE FOR AMPHOTERICIN B

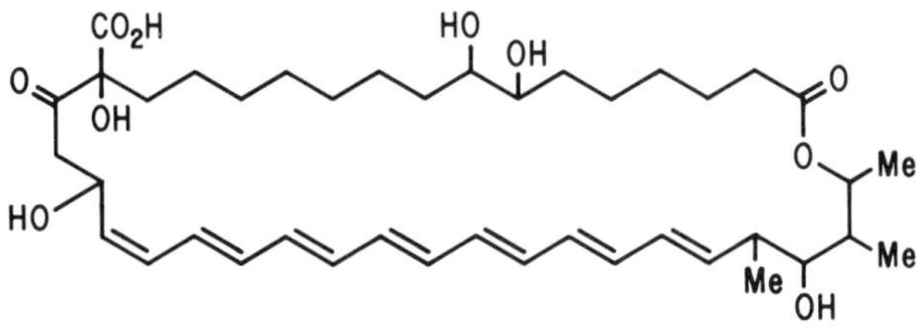

Figure 1–13. Amphotericin B is called a polyene because it contains a series of carbon atoms with multiple conjugated double bonds.

MYCOSAMINE

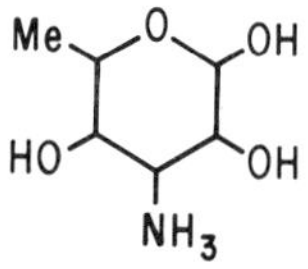

Figure 1–14. This amino sugar, mycosamine, is linked to a polyene in both amphotericin B and nystatin.

mine (Fig. 1–13), which is not present in many of the polyenes that are unsuitable for medical use.[3] Their extensive unsaturation makes them unstable compounds, especially in acid or alkaline solutions. They are also unstable in light and air. Although the exact formula has not been worked out for either one, amphotericin B is known to be a conjugated heptaene lactone linked with mycosamine and has the tentative formula $C_{46}H_{73}O_{20}N$ (Fig. 1–14).

SYNTHETIC ANTIMICROBIAL DRUGS

The Sulfonamides

The term "sulfonamide" refers to derivatives of sulfanilamide, or p-aminobenzenesulfonamide (Fig. 1–15), the first antimicrobial shown to be effective systemically for the treatment of human bacterial infection.[10] Thousands of sulfonamides have been synthesized, but only a dozen are of value for patients.

Most derivatives are made by substitutions on the sulfonamide group (SO_2NH_2), since these increase the antimicrobial activity. The para-NH_2 group, on the other hand, must remain free, or become free, after hydrolysis. Succinylsulfathiazole (Sulfasuxidine) is a good example of how the para-NH_2 group becomes free after slow hydrolysis from its inactive form to the active sulfathiazole. The substitutions on the SO_2NH_2 group of other sulfonamides are shown in Figure 1–15.

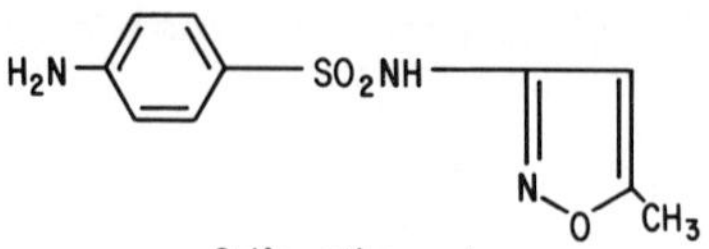

Sulfamethoxazole

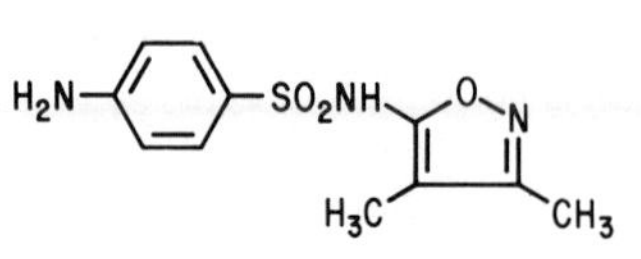

Sulfisoxazole, U.S.P.

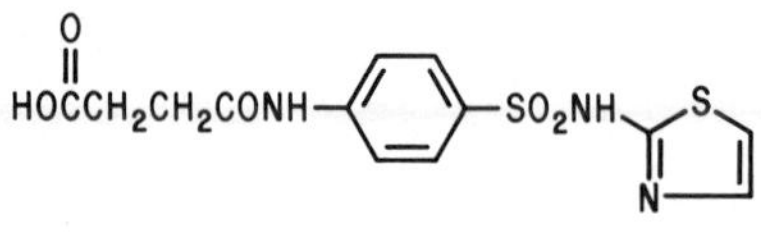

Succinylsulfathiazole, U.S.P.

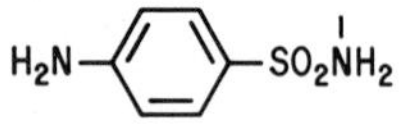

Sulfanilamide

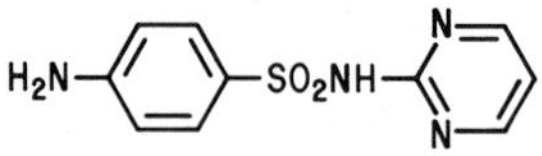

Sulfadiazine, U.S.P.

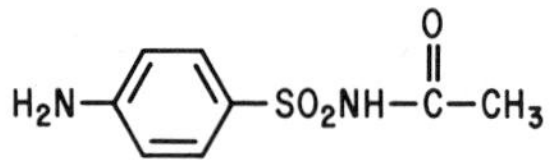

Sulfacetamide

Figure 1–15. These and other sulfonamide derivatives are made by substitutions on the SO_2NH_2 group of the parent compound sulfanilamide. The para-NH_2 group must remain free.

The Sulfones

As is evident from the structural formula of dapsone in Figure 1–16, sulfones are related to sulfonamides but lack the sulfonamide group and its broad antibacterial spectrum. Instead, the sulfones are limited in antibacterial activity to the leprosy bacillus.

Isoniazid and Ethionamide

Isoniazid was the first modern chemotherapeutic agent synthesized (1912), but its value in tuberculosis was not appreciated until 1952.[4] It is the hydrazide of isonicotinic acid (Fig. 1–17). Ethionamide is also a derivative of isonicotinic acid.

The Diaminopyrimidines

The diaminopyrimidine compounds were first synthesized as analogues of the nitrogenous bases found in DNA. Pyrimethamine, for example, was prepared as a thymine analogue. This drug and trimethoprim are the only two members of this group that are of practical medical impor-

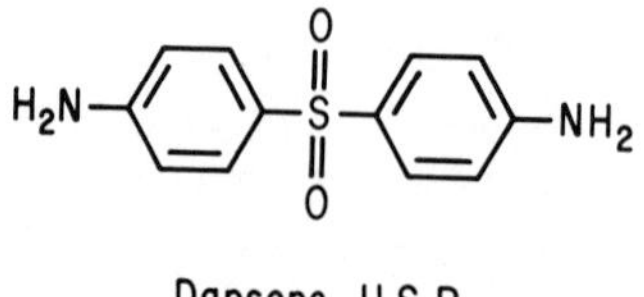

Dapsone, U.S.P.

Figure 1–16. Note structural relationship of dapsone to sulfonamides.

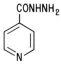

Figure 1–17. The drug isoniazid is a derivative of isonicotinic acid.

ISONIAZID

tance. Their formulas are given in Figure 1–18. Both are useful in protozoal infections, and trimethoprim shows promise in bacterial infections.[7]

The Fluorinated Pyrimidines

The substitution of fluorine for hydrogen in the 5-position on pyrimidines was first made in order to produce the pyrimidine analogue, 5-fluorouracil, a potent antimetabolite for mammalian cells and useful in cancer chemotherapy. Another fluorinated pyrimidine, 5-fluorocytosine (5FC), does not seem to be metabolized in mammalian cells and has no activity against cancer cells. The activity of 5FC against microorganisms seems to be related to its conversion to 5-fluorouracil by deamination[9] (Fig. 1–19).

The Nitrofurans

The nitrofurans are derivatives of the 5-membered ring sugars known as furans and possess a nitro group in the 5-position. The chief nitrofuran available for clinical application is shown in Figure 1–20 and is the only sugar derivative with clinically important antibacterial properties.

The Aminoquinolines

The most important member of the aminoquinolines is chloroquine, a 4-aminoquinoline with the structure shown in Figure 1–21. The main parts

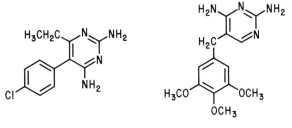

Pyrimethamine   Trimethoprim

Figure 1–18. These diaminopyrimidines were first synthesized as analogues of the nitrogenous bases found in DNA.

DEAMINATION OF 5-FLUOROCYTOSINE TO 5-FLUOROURACIL

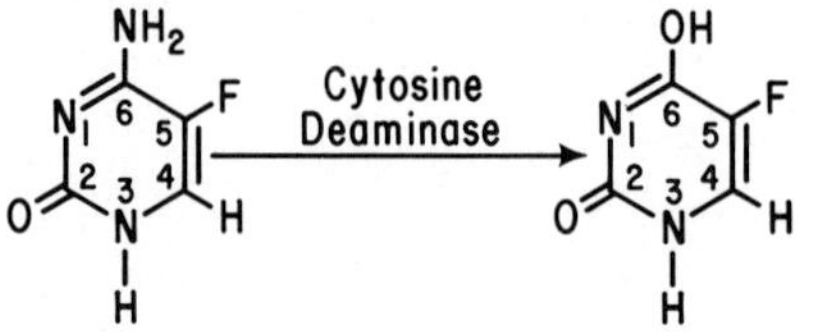

5-Fluorocytosine   5-Fluorouracil

Figure 1–19. The activity of 5-fluorocytosine against microorganisms seems to be related to its conversion to 5-fluorouracil.

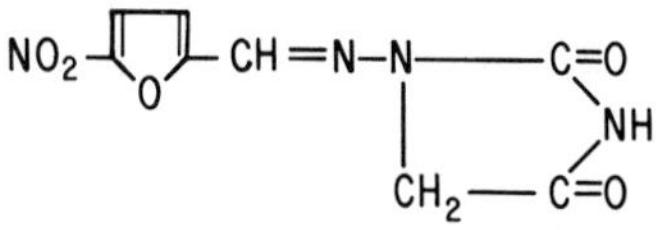

FURADANTIN

Figure 1–20. The nitrofurans are the only synthetic sugar derivatives with clinically useful antibacterial properties.

Figure 1–21. The Cl atom in position 7 is necessary for maximum antimalarial activity of chloroquine.

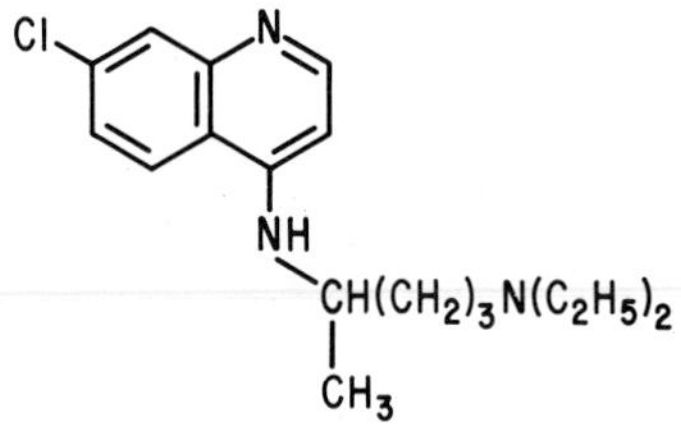

Chloroquine

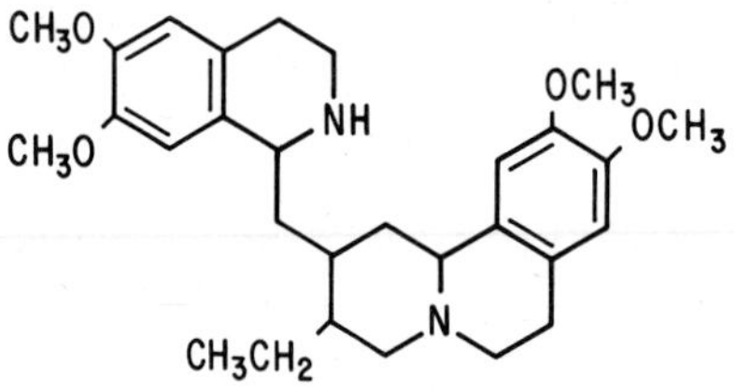

Figure 1–22. Emetine. This is the structure of the active principle of ipecac.

EMETINE

Figure 1–23. Piperazine has the simplest structure of the anthelmintics.

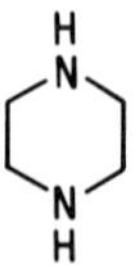

PIPERAZINE

of the molecule are the quinoline nucleus composed of a double ring and the alkyl side chain. The chlorine atom in position 7 of the quinoline nucleus appears necessary for maximum antimalarial activity.

Although first used as an antimalarial, chloroquine was later found to be valuable in the treatment of amebic liver abscess and giardiasis.

Emetine

Emetine is the oldest amebicidal drug and the active principle chiefly responsible for the clinical efficacy of ipecac in amebic infections. Emetine hydrochloride is obtained from ipecac as a hydrated hydrochloride[5] (Fig. 1–22).

Metronidazole

Metronidazole is the newest amebicidal drug. It is a nitroimidazole derivative, and its activity against amebae is possibly due to the reduction of the nitro group to a nitrosohydroxylamino group, which is more reactive. Metronidazole is also useful in the treatment of giardiasis, fusospirochetal infections of the mouth, and perhaps other anaerobic infections. The key to its activity may be that these organisms in the mouth and bowel, including the pathogenic protozoa, are all anaerobes.

The Anthelmintics[2]

The simplest structure of the anthelmintics, a group of nitro ring compounds, is that of piperazine, a drug used unsuccessfully at first for the treatment of gout but later found to be highly effective against *Ascaris* and *Enterobius* worms. Modification of piperazine (Fig. 1–23) by substituting a

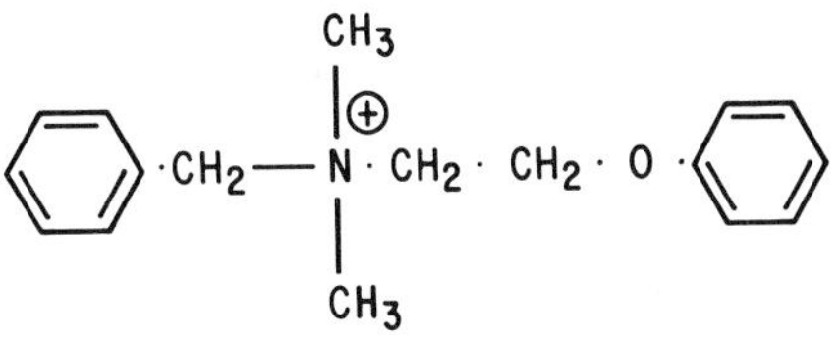

BEPHENIUM

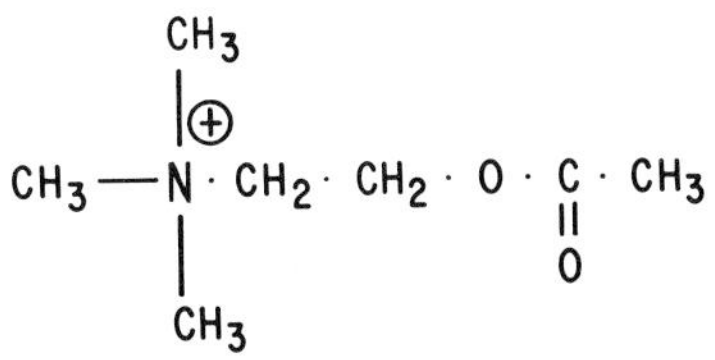

ACETYLCHOLINE

Figure 1–24. The anthelmintic bephenium resembles acetylcholine in structure and action. Bephenium paralyzes nematodes by causing membrane depolarization of muscle in the worms.

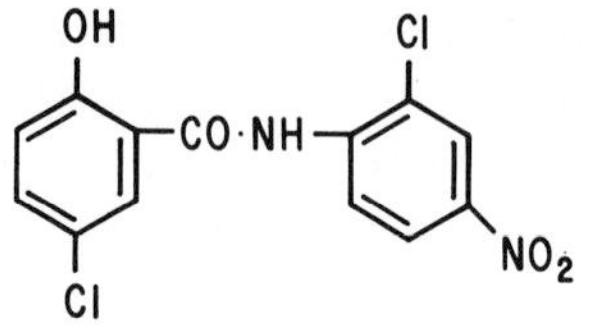

Figure 1–25. Niclosamide resembles in structure desaspidin, the active principle of oleoresin of aspidium, an old remedy for tapeworms.

NICLOSAMIDE

Figure 1–26. Thiabendazole is the best anthelmintic among several hundred substituted benzimidazole compounds.

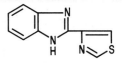

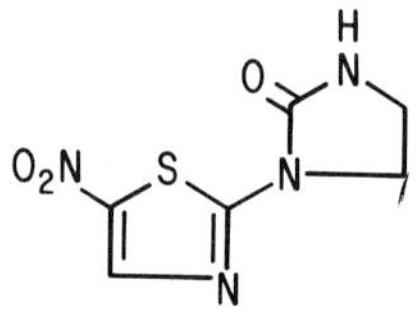

Thiabendazole

Figure 1–27. Niridazole. Note structural similarity of this anthelmintic to the antibacterial drug nitrofurantoin.

NIRIDAZOLE

diethylcarbamyl group at the 1-position and a methyl group at the 4-position created diethylcarbamazine, a drug that can kill adult filaria and microfilaria. Bephenium is a quaternary amine and resembles acetylcholine in both structure and function (Fig. 1–24). The anticestodal drug, niclosamide (chlorsalicylamide), resembles closely the structure of desaspidin, the active principle of oleoresin of aspidium, the oldest remedy for tapeworms (Fig. 1–25). Another important group of anthelmintics are the substituted benzimidazole compounds. One of these, thiabendazole, is effective against various round worms, while mebendazole is the only anthelmintic effective against both tapeworms and round worms. The formula of thiabendazole is shown in Figure 1–26. The only compound with a close structural resemblance to antibacterial drugs is niridazole, which is derived from a nitrothiazole nucleus (Fig. 1–27). Its structure is related to that of nitrofurantoin and metronidazole, two agents with antibacterial activity.

REFERENCES

1. Bodanszky M, Perlman D: Peptide antibiotics. Science *163*:352–358, 1969.
2. Bueding E: Some biochemical effects of anthelmintic drugs. Biochem Pharmacol *18*:1541–1547, 1969.
3. Dutcher JD, Young MB, Sherman JH, et al: Chemical studies on amphotericin B. I. Preparation of the hydrogenation product and isolation of mycosamine, an acetolysis product. Antibiot Annu 866–869, 1956–1957.
4. Fox H: The chemical attack on tuberculosis. Trans NY Acad Sci *15*:234–242, 1953.

5. Grollman P: Structural basis for inhibition of protein synthesis by emetine and cycloheximide based on an analogy between ipecac alkaloids and glutarimide antibiotics. Proc Nat Acad Sci USA 56:1867–1874, 1966.
6. Hewitt L: The cephalosporins—1973. J Infect Dis 128:Suppl:S312–319, 1973.
7. Hitchings H: Species differences among dihydrofolate reductases as a basis for chemotherapy. Postgrad Med J 45:Suppl:7–10, 1969.
8. Johnson A, Anker H, Meleney L: Bacitracin; new antibiotic produced by member of B. subtilis group. Science 102:376–377, 1945.
9. Lacroute F: Regulation of pyrimidine biosynthesis in Saccharomyces cerevisiae. J Bacteriol 95:824–832, 1968.
10. Long H, Bliss A: Para-amino-benzene-sulfonamide and its derivatives; experimental and clinical observations on their use in treatment of beta-hemolytic streptococcic infection: preliminary report. JAMA 108:32–37, 1937.
11. Novick P: Staphylococcal penicillinase and the new penicillins. Biochem J 83:229–235, 1962.
12. Oxford E, Raistrick H, Simonart P: XXIX. Studies in the biochemistry of microorganisms: LX. Griseofulvin, $C_{17}H_{17}O_6Cl$, a metabolic product of Penicillium griseofulvum Dierckx. Biochem J 33:240–248, 1939.
13. Wehrli W, Staehelin M: Actions of the rifamycins. Bacteriol Rev 35:290–309, 1971.

CHAPTER 2

MECHANISMS OF ACTION

The key to antibiotic action is a selective toxicity for the infecting organism but not for the patient. Antibiotics can hit at least four targets in bacteria and other organisms that are either missing or less vulnerable in human cells: the cell wall, the cytoplasmic membrane, the ribosomes, and the molecules involved in transcription of genetic information.

CELL WALL

The cell wall is where the penicillins and cephalosporins do their damage. It is the most important target for antibiotics because it is absent in human cells. The cell wall of bacteria is a thick rigid envelope that surrounds the cell membrane, maintaining the shape of the bacteria and keeping them from osmotic damage in water and body fluids. The internal pressures of pathogenic bacteria are somewhat higher than serum and other extracellular fluids so that the organisms would imbibe water, swell, and burst if the cell

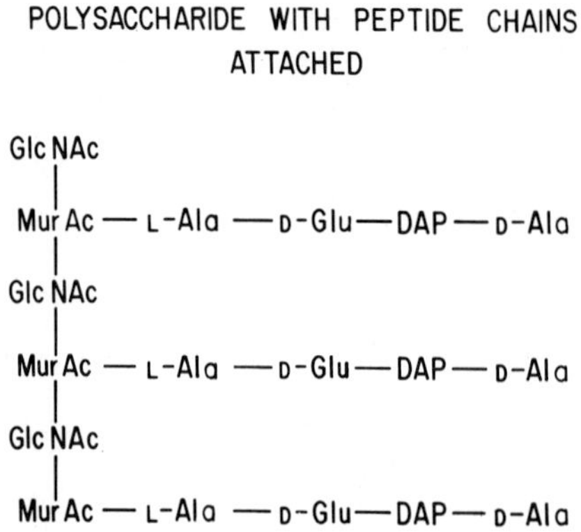

POLYSACCHARIDE WITH PEPTIDE CHAINS
ATTACHED

GlcNAc
|
MurAc — L-Ala — D-Glu—DAP — D-Ala
|
GlcNAc
|
MurAc — L-Ala — D-Glu—DAP — D-Ala
|
GlcNAc
|
MurAc — L-Ala — D-Glu—DAP — D-Ala

Figure 2–1. The rigid structure in bacterial cell walls is a sugar peptide called mucopeptide or murein. The sugar is a polysaccharide of muramic acid (MurAc) and glucosamine (GlcNAc). The peptides are composed of four amino acids: L-alanine (L-Ala), D-glutamic acid (D-Glu), α,ϵ-diaminopimelic acid (DAP), and D-alanine.

18

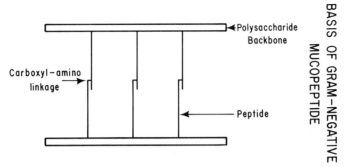

Figure 2–2. Cross linking of peptide chains in gram-negative bacilli by bonds between the free carboxyl groups of D-alanine and the NH_2 groups of α,ϵ-diaminopimelic acid. (Modified from Rogers HJ: The mode of action of antibiotics. *In* The Biological Basis of Medicine, Vol. 2. Edited by Bittar, EE. New York, Academic Press, 1968, p. 427.)

wall became defective. The rigid portion of the cell wall, known as the sacculus, is reminiscent of grape hulls in cocci and balloons in bacilli. The rigid material in the sacculus is a material composed of sugar and peptides and called mucopeptide or murein. The mucopeptide is at least four times thicker in gram-positive cells than in gram-negative cells. In *E. coli* the layer of mucopeptide is made up of polysaccharide chains linked together by peptides. The polysaccharide chains are composed of repeating units of two sugars, muramic acid and N-acetylglucosamine, as indicated in Figure 2–1. The cross-linking peptide strands are attached to the polysaccharide chains by a peptide bond between the carboxyl group in each muramic acid unit and the amino group of L-alanine. Another peptide bond connects L-alanine to D-glutamic acid, followed in turn by α,ϵ-diaminopimelic acid, and finally D-alanine to form a tetrapeptide. The free carboxyl groups on the D-alanine residues are also attached to the NH_2 group of the α,ϵ-diaminopimelic acid in adjacent tetrapeptides to produce a cross-linked structure (Fig. 2–2). In staphylococci a second chain composed of five glycine molecules is used to

STAPHYLOCOCCAL MUCOPEPTIDE

Figure 2–3. In staphylococci a second chain composed of 5-glycine (pentaglycine) molecules connects the neighboring peptides. (Modified from Rogers HJ: The mode of action of antibiotics. *In* The Biological Basis of Medicine, Vol. 2. Edited by Bittar, EE. New York, Academic Press, 1968, p. 428.)

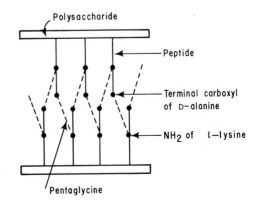

connect neighboring peptides so that the structure is more like that in Figure 2–3. The peptide group in staphylococci is also different from that in *E. coli*, as shown in Figure 2–4. The staphylococcal peptide lacks diaminopimelic acid and, instead, has L-lysine as the third amino acid. This is followed by D-alanyl-D-alanine at the end of the chain. The murein network in the *Staphylococcus* is completed when D-alanine is split from D-alanyl-D-alanine so that a peptide bond can form between the carboxyl group of the residual D-alanine and the terminal amino group of the pentaglycine chain (Fig. 2–4).

Penicillin is thought to act by preventing the final peptide bond between D-alanine and glycine.[26] It has been suggested that penicillin combines with the enzyme responsible for this final cross linkage (the cross-linking enzyme). Since the stearic configuration of penicillin is like that of D-alanyl-D-alanine, penicillin might react with the cross-linking enzyme and inactivate it so that it could not complete the transpeptidation reaction (Fig. 2–5).

An important feature of penicillin action is its ability to kill growing bacterial cells, but not stationary organisms. During growth, hydrolases produce gaps in the mucopeptide that are filled with new structural units. These units are tied into the mucopeptide by the transpeptidation (cross-linking) reaction and can therefore be blocked by penicillin so that open gaps

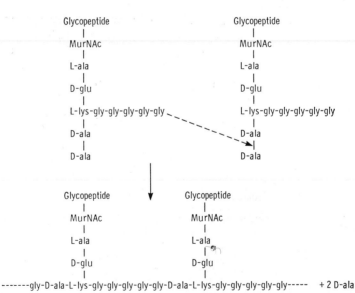

Figure 2–4. Mucopeptide from staphylococci. The peptide chain differs from that in *E. coli* (Fig. 2–1) in that staphylococcal peptide lacks diaminopimelic acid and instead has L-lysine as the third amino acid. The murein network is completed when D-alanine is split from D-alanyl-D-alanine so that a peptide bond can form between the carboxyl group of the residual D-alanine and the terminal group of the pentaglycine chain. Penicillin is thought to act by inhibiting the enzyme (transpeptidase) responsible for this cross linkage. (From Strominger JL: Enzymatic reactions in bacterial cell wall synthesis sensitive to penicillins and other antibacterial substances. *In* Microbial Protoplasts, Spheroplasts and L-Forms. Edited by Guze LB. Baltimore, The Williams & Wilkins Co., 1968, p. 57.)

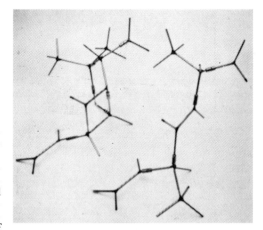

Figure 2–5. Stereomodels of penicillin (left) and the end of the peptide D-alanyl-D-alanine have suggested that penicillin is a structural analogue of the D-alanyl-D-alanine end of the peptide and thereby can react with the transpeptidase to prevent the transpeptidation reaction required for closure of the glycine bridges between peptide chains. (From Strominger JL: Enzymatic reactions in bacterial cell wall synthesis sensitive to penicillins and other antibacterial substances. *In* Microbial Protoplasts, Spheroplasts and L-Forms. Edited by Guze LB. Baltimore, The Williams & Wilkins Co., 1968, p. 58.)

remain in the mucopeptide. The cell membrane extends through these gaps and ruptures under osmotic stress, and the cell dies (Fig. 2–6). Cells that are not undergoing multiplication can survive in the presence of penicillin because their mucopeptide is unbroken and there is no reparative cross-linking activity for the penicillin to block. These cells are known as "persisters" and may be responsible for recurrence of infection after penicillin treatment has been stopped.[11] All penicillin and cephalosporin derivatives kill bacteria by the same mechanism.

While penicillins block the terminal cross-linking reaction of mucopeptide formation, it is also theoretically possible for antibiotics to prevent the synthesis or transfer of mucopeptide precursors. Such action against precursors by certain antibiotics does, in fact, take place, but these are of minor clinical importance. Cycloserine is a structural analogue of D-alanine and competitively inhibits the enzyme responsible for synthesis of D-alanyl-D-alanine, an essential component of the pentapeptide.[19] Bacitracin[25] and vancomycin[1] both block the stages of cell wall construction which

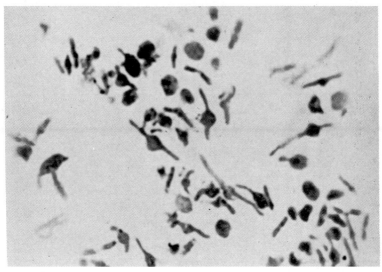

Figure 2–6. Effect of penicillin on cell wall of gram-negative bacilli. Defective portions of the mucopeptide allow the high internal osmotic pressure to cause swellings in both the central and terminal portions of the rods. (From Braude AI, Siemienski J, Jacobs I: Protoplast formation in human urine. Trans Assoc Am Physicians 74:238, 1961, Fig. 3.)

involve the transfer of the sugar pentapeptide from the site of synthesis in the cytoplasm to its attachment to a lipid in the cell membrane.

CYTOPLASMIC MEMBRANE

Beneath the rigid cell wall is a membrane that totally encloses the cytoplasm (Fig. 2–7A). This cytoplasmic membrane resembles that of human cells in possessing lipid and protein structural elements. Bacterial lipids are mainly phospholipids. Fungi contain sterols in their membranes that are not present in bacteria.

The lipoproteins in the cytoplasmic membrane of all cells account for selective permeability to water, ions, and nutrients. The polymyxins are cationic detergents that react with the phosphate groups of cell envelope phospholipids and disorganize the lipoproteins in the bacterial cytoplasmic membrane by inserting the lipophilic portion of their molecule into the membrane lipid. This causes leakage of amino acids, purines, pyrimidines, and other small molecules from inside the cell so that nucleic acids and proteins break down and the cell dies.[10, 20]

Amphotericin and other polyene antibiotics also alter the permeability of sensitive cells, but only in organisms whose membranes contain sterols. For this reason they do not affect bacteria and are limited in their action against pathogenic organisms to yeasts, fungi (Fig. 2–7B), and certain amebae. After reacting with polyenes, sterols probably become reoriented within the membranes so that permeability is altered.[16]

RIBOSOMES

Ribosomes act as an assembly line where amino acids are strung together into peptide chains and proteins. The process is directed by messenger RNA (mRNA), which carries the code for protein synthesis from nuclear DNA. The message in the code is *transcribed* from DNA to RNA (Fig. 2–8A) and translated into the appropriate amino acid sequence by the four types of ribonucleotides in mRNA. These four ribonucleotides are prearranged in 4^3 (or 64) different triplet combinations that are able to specify different amino acids. Since there are 64 triplets and only 20 amino acids used in protein synthesis, many amino acids are selected by more than one triplet (or codon). Three of the codons (UAA, UAG, and UGA) code for chain termination only and do not select amino acids. Each amino acid specified by the triplet is carried to the ribosome for incorporation into the growing peptide chain by a second type of RNA, transfer RNA (tRNA).

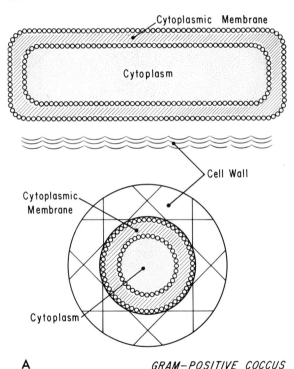

GRAM–NEGATIVE BACILLUS

Cytoplasmic Membrane

Cytoplasm

Cell Wall

Cytoplasmic Membrane

Cytoplasm

A   GRAM–POSITIVE COCCUS

Figure 2–7. A, Bacterial cell wall and underlying cytoplasmic membrane. The circles indicate the protein, and the adjacent diagonal lines represent the lipid in the lipoprotein cytoplasmic membrane. The cytoplasmic membrane is drawn out of proportion to its true relationship to the rest of the cell for purposes of illustration. In gram-negative bacilli the cytoplasmic membrane is the site of action of the polymyxins, but in gram-positive cocci it is not damaged by those drugs in usual doses. Differences in accessibility to the membrane, related to differences in cell wall, may account for these differences in susceptibility between gram-positive and gram-negative organisms.

Illustration continued on the following page.

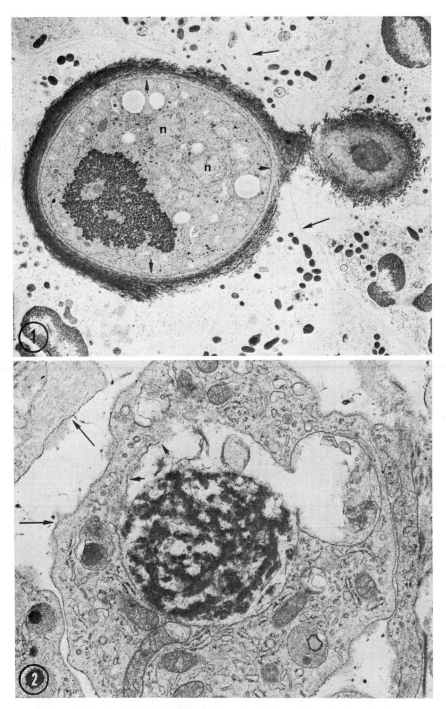

Figure 2–7B, 1 and 2. *Legend and illustration continued on the opposite page.*

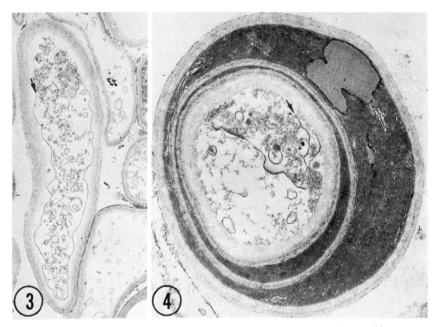

Figure 2–7 Continued. *B,* Effect of amphotericin B on cytoplasmic membrane of fungi. 1, 2, 3, and 4 show *in vivo* effect of amphotericin during treatment of human North American blastomycosis. (Courtesy Dr. Henry C. Powell.)

1. Skin biopsy, North American blastomycosis. Budding organism: the parent cell shows two nuclei (n), numerous mitochondria, and aggregates of electron-dense material (probably glycogen) enclosed by the cell membrane (arrowheads) and the rough outer coat. The surfaces of surrounding macrophages are closely apposed (arrows). ×20,000. 2. Skin biopsy, North American blastomycosis, after amphotericin treatment. Rupture of the cell membrane (arrowhead) and cytolysis. ×20,000. 3. North American blastomycosis. Fungal cells *in vitro* after incubation with amphotericin and 5-fluorocytosine. Note lysis of the cell membranes (arrow) and cytoplasmic degeneration. ×7000. 4. Degenerating fungal cell with electron-dense deposits in the cell wall. ×20,000.

The triplet AUG (adenylyl-uridylyl-guanylyl) or GUG initiates peptide chain formation by directing tRNA carrying methionine (as N-formyl-methionine) to attach to the ribosome.

The bacterial ribosomes are spherical particles with a molecular weight of nearly 3 million. They sediment in the Svedberg ultracentrifuge at a rate expressed as 70S (Svedberg units). Before protein synthesis is started, the ribosome dissociates into a 30S subunit and a 50S subunit (Fig. 2–8*B*). Protein synthesis starts when mRNA attaches to the 30S subunit and tRNA carrying methionine is bound (Fig. 2–8*C*). This is followed by recombination with the 50S subunit to form the functioning 70S ribosome (Fig. 2–8*D*). The complete 70S ribosome has another binding site for tRNA, so that a second tRNA molecule carrying another amino acid becomes attached (Fig. 2–8*E*, step 1). The first amino acid (methionine) is linked to the second amino acid by the enzyme, peptidyltransferase, the two being joined by a

DNA

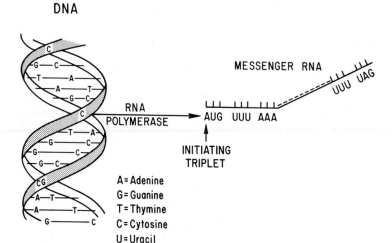

A = Adenine
G = Guanine
T = Thymine
C = Cytosine
U = Uracil

A. Transcription

Figure 2–8. *A,* Messenger RNA receives the code for amino acid sequence (and thus protein synthesis) from DNA in a process known as transcription. The message is carried to the ribosomes in the form of nucleotide triplets. Since there are four nucleotides in mRNA, they can be arranged in 4^3 or 64 different triplet combinations, and each can specify one of the 20 amino acids. As each triplet reaches the ribosome it directs the attachment of a specific amino acid. Rifampin, chloroquine, 5-iodo-2′-deoxyuridine, 5-fluorocytosine, sulfonamides, pyrimethamine, and trimethoprim all interfere with transcription by one or more mechanisms as described in the text.

peptide bond between the carboxyl group of formylmethionine and the amino group of the second amino acid (Fig. 2–8E, step 2). This beginning chain with its tRNA is translocated to the first site (donor site) after it has been vacated by the release of tRNA that had formerly carried formylmethionine (Fig. 2–8E, steps 3 and 4). The ribosome then moves along the chain of mRNA to the next

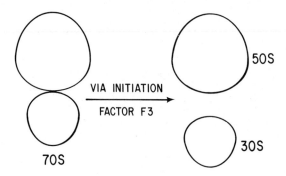

B. Dissociation of 70S ribosome

Figure 2–8 Continued. *B,* Dissociation of the 70S ribosome is the first step in protein synthesis on ribosomes.

Illustration continued on the opposite page.

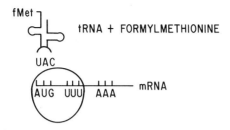

C. Formation of initiation complex
between mRNA, fMet and tRNA

Figure 2–8 Continued. *C*, Protein synthesis starts when mRNA attaches to the 30S subunit and then tRNA + formylmethionine are bound. The 50S subunit then reassociates and the initiation complex is completed. Streptomycin binds the 30S subunit and inactivates the initiation complex so that it cannot form peptide bonds. The tetracyclines also bind to the 30S subunit and prevent binding of tRNA.

triplet codon for further instruction. Here directions are given for the attachment to the unoccupied acceptor site of a third tRNA with its amino acid. The dipeptide on the donor site is transferred to the third amino acid, and the process of chain elongation is continued until a termination code triplet in mRNA announces that the protein chain is complete.

Since the mRNA strand is "read" by several ribosomes simultaneously, multiple proteins are synthesized simultaneously. A connecting mRNA fiber between adjacent ribosomes, which forms an assembly of as many as 100 ribosomes on a single mRNA strand, can be seen in the electron microscope. This arrangement of multiple ribosomes, each producing its own protein, is called a polyribosome.

Antibiotics that bind to ribosomes cure infections by interfering at certain points with peptide chain formation in bacteria. Thus, they may interfere with initiation of the peptide chain, the attachment of tRNA after initiation, peptide-bond formation, translocation, and the movement of

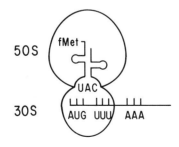

D. Reassociation of 50S and 30S
subunits to form functional 70S
ribosome

Figure 2–8 Continued. *D*, Reassociation of 50S and 30S subunits to form functional 70S ribosome.

Illustration continued on the following page.

ribosomes along mRNA. Among antimicrobials important in clinical medicine, the mechanism of such interference has been worked out best for five groups: the aminoglycosides, the tetracyclines, chloramphenicol, erythromycin, and emetine.

ELONGATION (GROWTH) OF PEPTIDE

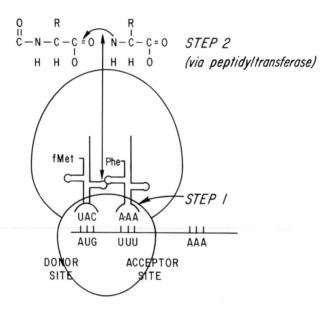

STEP 1: Binding of tRNA + 2nd amino acid (e.g. phenylalanine) to acceptor site of 70S ribosome, as directed by 2nd triplet on mRNA (e.g. UUU).

STEP 2: Formation of peptide bond by reaction of amino group of newly bound amino acid (e.g. phenylalanine) with carboxyl group of methionine. The enzyme peptidyltransferase in the 50S subunit catalyzes this reaction.

E

Figure 2–8 Continued. E, Step 1: The second amino acid is brought in by tRNA after the initiation complex is completed. Step 2: This binds the two amino acids by a peptide bond and is blocked by chloramphenicol and lincomycin.

Illustration continued on the opposite page.

The Aminoglycosides

The mode of action of streptomycin has been examined far more than that of other aminoglycosides. Streptomycin binds to the 30S subunit of the ribosome by irreversibly combining with a specific ribosomal protein, designated P10. At this site it has three effects on protein synthesis: (1) It permits formation of the initiation complex but blocks its normal activity. When streptomycin attaches to ribosomes, they fall off the "assembly line"; i.e., they leave mRNA prematurely. These ribosomes dissociate into 30S and 50S subunits which subsequently reassociate at the normal initiation sites on mRNA, but they remain irreversibly inactivated initiation com-

ELONGATION OF PEPTIDE

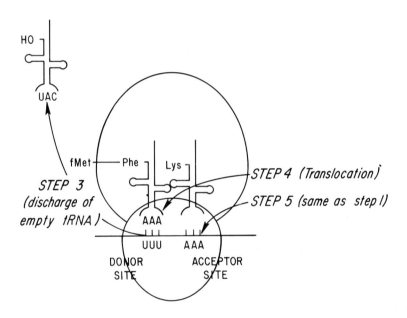

STEP 3: Discharge of empty tRNA (formerly carrying formylmethionine) from donor site on 70S ribosome.

STEP 4: Translocation of mRNA and tRNA with new peptide bond (between methionine and e.g. phenylalanine) to donor site on 70S ribosome.

E

Figure 2–8 Continued. *E,* Steps 3 and 4: The first tRNA is ejected from the ribosome and the second tRNA with its dipeptide is translocated to the site vacated by the first tRNA. The ribosome then moves along the chain of mRNA to the next triplet codon for instruction on the identity of the third amino acid to be introduced into the growing peptide chain. Erythromycin blocks the translocation step.

plexes that cannot form peptide bonds. (2) It interferes with the attachment of tRNA. (3) It distorts the triplet codons of mRNA so that the message is misread, the wrong amino acids are inserted into the peptide chain, and faulty proteins are produced. Of these three effects, the first is the most important cause of bacterial killing by streptomycin. Cells are killed by the accumulation of aberrant inactive initiation complexes.[17, 21] The third occurs only at borderline inhibitory concentrations of streptomycin.[6]

Other aminoglycosides such as kanamycin, neomycin, and gentamicin probably act similarly, but more research is necessary to establish their mode of action.

The Tetracyclines

These drugs also bind to the 30S subunit of bacterial ribosomes and block the binding of tRNA to the mRNA 30S ribosomal subunit.[5] In other words, tetracyclines prevent the introduction of new amino acids into the peptide chain so that protein synthesis cannot proceed.

Chloramphenicol

In contrast to the aminoglycosides and tetracyclines, chloramphenicol attaches exclusively to the larger (50S) moiety of the ribosome. The drug prevents peptide-bond formation by inhibiting the enzyme peptidyltransferase. This enzyme is located in the 50S subunit, so that it is blocked when chloramphenicol binds to that portion of the ribosome.[22]

Erythromycin

Like chloramphenicol, erythromycin binds to 50S ribosomal subunits and can compete with chloramphenicol for binding sites on 50S ribosomes. Like chloramphenicol, it interferes with peptidyltransferase activity.[18]

Lincomycin

This antibiotic resembles erythromycin in its antibacterial spectrum and also acts like chloramphenicol in inhibiting protein synthesis. Thus, lincomycin binds to 50S ribosomes (but not ribosomes of E. coli, organisms whose growth is not inhibited by lincomycin) and also appears to block the peptidyltransferase reaction necessary for peptide-bond formation.

Emetine

This ancient amebicidal drug has only recently been found to be an inhibitor of protein synthesis. It inhibits the transfer of amino acids from tRNA to the polypeptide on the ribosome and prevents elongation, rather than initiation, of peptide chains. Emetine also inhibits protein synthesis in bacteria and mammalian cells. This lack of selectivity may explain the toxicity of emetine for patients during treatment of amebic dysentery or liver abscess.[12]

The Thiosemicarbazones (Methisazone)

If polyribosomes are disrupted, protein synthesis stops. At least one group of antimicrobials, the thiosemicarbazones, seem to interfere with protein synthesis of smallpox virus by breaking up the mRNA into smaller fragments and disrupting the ribosomes.[2]

TRANSCRIPTION MECHANISMS

The information that determines the sequence of amino acids in a given protein is coded in the DNA and *transcribed* into messenger RNA (see Fig. 2–8A). Messenger RNA then becomes attached to ribosomes, where the code is translated into protein synthesis. Antibiotics interfering with translation act on the ribosomes, as described in the preceding section. Drugs acting on transcription may interfere either with separation of DNA strands or with the synthesis of RNA. DNA consists of two polynucleotide chains twisted about each other in the form of a double helix. During transcription these strands of the double helix separate, and one of them serves as a specific surface or *template* upon which a complementary strand of RNA is synthesized through the action of RNA polymerase. The complementary RNA strand and its template DNA differ in only two respects: the presence of deoxyribose in DNA in place of ribose, and of thymine, in place of uracil, as one of the four major bases.

A drug can interfere with the transcription process by preventing strand separation of DNA, by breaking a strand, by introducing an improper component into the replicating RNA strand, or by blocking access of RNA polymerase to the template strand. Only one clinically valuable antibiotic, rifampicin, interferes with transcription. Other antimicrobial drugs, however, active against protozoa, fungi, and viruses act by interfering with transcription.

Rifampicin

This antibiotic is the most potent inhibitor of DNA-dependent RNA polymerase in bacteria. Human DNA-dependent RNA polymerase, on the other hand, is resistant to rifampicin, so that the drug is selectively toxic for bacterial but not human cells. By binding to RNA polymerase, rifampicin inhibits the formation of all forms of RNA in bacteria.[28]

Chloroquine

This important antiprotozoal drug inhibits nucleic acid synthesis by interfering with the ability of DNA to act as a template.[13] Chloroquine is inserted (intercalated) between the stacked base pairs of the double helix. This drug inhibits nucleic acid synthesis in mammalian cells as well, but protozoa concentrate chloroquine so that their intracellular level is much higher than that in the body fluids of the patient.

5-Iodo-2' deoxyuridine (IUDR)

This nucleoside analogue is widely used in the treatment of herpes simplex infections of the cornea. The drug is incorporated into *viral* DNA instead of thymidine.[15] Normally, deoxuridilic acid is converted to thymidilic acid by the enzyme, thymidilic acid synthetase. IUDR inhibits this enzyme so that insufficient thymidine phosphate is available for DNA synthesis. Strands of DNA containing IUDR in place of thymidine are more easily broken. In addition, the presence of IUDR in DNA could lead to abnormal base pairing and the consequent production of nonfunctional proteins that are not assembled into virus particles.[2]

5-Fluorocytosine

Like IUDR, this halogenated (fluorinated) pyrimidine probably acts by eventually inhibiting the action of the enzyme thymidilic acid synthetase. Cytosine is first deaminated to uracil by cytosine deaminase. 5-Fluorouracil is then converted to 5-fluorodeoxyuridylate. This fluorinated compound causes a lethal thymine deficiency by blocking the conversion of the normal deoxyribonucleotides to deoxythymidylate by thymidylate synthetase. 5-Fluorouracil is also incorporated into mRNA so that errors are produced in translation of information from DNA into protein.[7]

The Sulfonamides

This group of drugs is placed here among transcription inhibitors because sulfonamides block the synthesis of thymidine and all purines. Thymidine is necessary for DNA synthesis, and the purines for nucleic acid synthesis. This action of sulfonamides is accomplished by preventing the synthesis of folic acid (pteroylglutamic acid) by microbial cells. Sulfonamides are structural analogues of para-aminobenzoic acid (PABA), an essential ingredient of folic acid (Fig. 2–9). Competitive inhibition of PABA utilization by sulfonamides interferes with folic acid synthesis. Since folic acid functions as a coenzyme for transporting 1-carbon units from one molecule to another, the sulfonamides block these reactions which are necessary for the synthesis of thymidine, purines, methionine, and serine. Folic acid metabolism in patients is not affected by sulfonamides because human cells cannot synthesize folic acid. Instead, patients must obtain folic acid in their diets. Since bacteria cannot transport exogenous folic acid into their cells, dietary folate does not interfere with the action of sulfonamide drugs. In pus, however, the breakdown of cells may cause a considerable accumulation of thymidine, purines, methionine, and serine which reverse

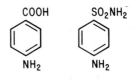

Figure 2-9. The close structural relationship of sulfonamides to para-aminobenzoic acid (PABA) is used to explain their antibacterial effect. The competitive inhibition of PABA utilization by sulfonamides interferes with folic acid synthesis in bacteria but not in man.

Structural relationship between p-aminobenzoic acid (left) and sulfanilamide (right)

the inhibitory effect of sulfonamides on bacteria by replenishing the end products of folic acid metabolism. In this way, the sulfonamides may lose therapeutic effectiveness.[9]

In addition to the sulfonamides, para-aminosalicylic acid (PAS) and the sulfones (both active against certain mycobacteria) are PABA analogues and block folic acid synthesis by competitive inhibition.

The Diaminopyrimidines

Both pyrimethamine and trimethoprim, the two important members of this group, are folic acid antagonists ("antifols"). Their site of action is different from that of the sulfonamides, however. The diaminopyrimidines are structurally similar to the pteridine portion of dihydrofolate; therefore instead of blocking PABA utilization, they prevent the conversion of folic acid to tetrahydrofolic acid by depression of the enzyme dihydrofolic reductase, as indicated in the following reactions:

$$PABA \rightarrow \text{folic acid} \xrightarrow[\text{reductase}]{\text{folic}} \text{dihydrofolic acid} \xrightarrow[\text{reductase}]{\text{dihydrofolic}} \text{tetrahydrofolic acid } (H_4FA)$$

$$\text{Precursors} \xrightarrow{H_4FA} \text{components of nucleic acids}$$

The dihydrofolic acid reductase of protozoa and certain other pathogenic organisms is far more sensitive to trimethoprim than that of man, so that folic acid deficiency in patients given trimethoprim is not a serious problem.[14]

In order to take advantage of the two vulnerable metabolic sites in protozoa and other pathogens, the diaminopyrimidines are usually given in conjunction with sulfonamides. This combination has a much greater antifol action than a simple summation of the two, and, since the two sequential depression steps are present only in the parasite, the combination has markedly increased activity against infection without an increased toxicity for patients.

MECHANISM OF ACTION OF ANTHELMINTIC DRUGS

Chemotherapy for worms is based on physiologic damage rather than protein inhibition. This is because pathogenic worms are fully grown when treatment is needed. Drugs that interfere with growth through inhibition of protein synthesis can stop egg production, but egg production is not needed for worm survival.

Anthelmintics kill worms by blocking energy metabolism or by paralysis.[3] Pyrvinium and mebendazole, for example, interfere with energy metabolism by blocking uptake of glucose, while thiabendazole inhibits fumaric reductase, a key enzyme in fermentation of glucose.[27] Like other intestinal microflora, worms are anaerobic and do not have the enzymes that mammalian cells use for terminal oxidation of glucose.[23] In the generation of energy-rich phosphate during glucose metabolism in worms, electron transfer is characterized by the reduction of fumarate to succinate through the action of fumarate reductase, which serves as an electron carrier from flavoproteins to fumarate. In other words, fumarate, instead of O_2, becomes the ultimate electron acceptor in worms as in the following schema of electron transfer in worms and man:

Worms   Flavoprotein $\rightarrow$ fumaric reductase $\rightarrow$ fumarate

Man   Flavoprotein $\rightarrow$ cytochrome oxidase $\rightarrow$ O_2

This selective inhibition of fumaric reductase explains the toxicity of thiabendazole for worms, but not man.

TABLE 2–1. *Mechanisms of Action of Antimicrobial Drugs*

NATURE OF INJURY	ANTIMICROBIAL DRUG	MODE OF ACTION
Defective cell wall mucopeptide	Penicillins and cephalosporins	Prevent final peptide bond between D-alanine and glycine
	Cycloserine	As structural analogue of D-alanine, it inhibits enzymes responsible for synthesis of D-alanyl-D-alanine, an essential component of mucopeptide
	Bacitracin and vancomycin	Block transfer to cell membrane of sugar pentapeptide from site of synthesis in cytoplasm
Damaged cytoplasmic membrane	Polymyxins	Disorganize lipoproteins by inserting lipophobic moiety into membrane lipid
	Polyenes	React with steroids in fungal membranes so that permeability is altered
Impaired function of ribosomes	Aminoglycosides	Bind to 30S ribosomal unit, causing ribosomes to leave mRNA prematurely; also interfere with attachment of tRNA and distort triplet codons so that message is misread
	Tetracyclines	Bind to 30S unit and block binding of tRNA so that new amino acids cannot be introduced into peptide chain

Table continued on the opposite page.

Niclosamide, another important anthelmintic, interferes with energy metabolism by blocking the phosphorylation of adenosine diphosphate (ADP) and thus the formation of adenosine triphosphate (ATP) during electron transport. In other words, the high-energy phosphate required for energy by the worm is not generated in the presence of niclosamide. Niclosamide would, no doubt, show the same effect on human ATP formation, but fortunately the drug is not absorbed from the intestine.

TABLE 2–1 Continued. *Mechanisms of Action of Antimicrobial Drugs*

Nature of Injury	Antimicrobial Drug	Mode of Action
	Chloramphenicol	Attaches to 50S subunit of ribosomes and prevents peptide-bond formation by inhibiting enzyme peptidyltransferase
	Erythromycin and lincomycin	Same as chloramphenicol
	Emetine	Prevents elongation of peptide chain by inhibiting transfer of amino acids from tRNA to polypeptide on ribosome
	Thiosemicarbazones	Disrupt polyribosomes
Impaired nucleic acid function	Rifampicin	Blocks bacterial RNA formation by inhibiting DNA-dependent RNA polymerase
	Chloroquine	Inserted between stacked base pairs in double helix and thus interferes with ability of DNA to act as a template for nucleic acid synthesis
	5-Iodo-2′deoxyuridine	Incorporated into viral DNA instead of thymidine so that nonfunctional proteins are synthesized
	5-Fluorocytosine	Converted to 5-fluorouracil which blocks thymidylate synthetase so that lethal thymine deficiency results
	Sulfonamides and diaminopyrimidines	By preventing synthesis of folic acid, they block formation of thymidine and purines needed for nucleic acid synthesis
Impaired energy metabolism	Pyrvinium and mebendazole	Block glucose uptake
	Thiabendazole	Inhibits fumaric reductase so that glucose fermentation is impaired
	Niclosamide	Blocks phosphorylation of ATP
	Niridazole	Depletes glycogen reserves
Paralysis	Piperazine	Stabilizes membrane potential of *Ascaris* muscle by hyperpolarization
	Bephenium	Depolarizes membranes (i.e., reverse of piperazine)

Niridazole, a powerful new remedy for schistosomiasis, affects energy metabolism by depleting glycogen reserves. It blocks the inhibitor of glycogen phosphorylase so that glycogenolysis becomes excessive.[4]

Two important paralyzing anthelmintics are piperazine and bephenium hydroxynaphthoate.[24] Piperazine produces flaccid paralysis of *Ascaris* so that the worm can be expelled from the patient by intestinal peristalsis.[8] It stabilizes the membrane potential of *Ascaris* muscle by hyperpolarization, but has no effect on human muscle. Hence its toxicity is fully selective for the parasite. Bephenium, which resembles acetylcholine in structure and function, has the reverse effect on nematodes. Instead of hyperpolarization and flaccid paralysis, it causes depolarization and contraction. Since the cuticle of many worms is impervious to bephenium, the drug is effective against only a few nematodes of clinical importance, including *Necator americanus*, *Ancylostoma duodenale*, and *Ascaris lumbricoides*. The mucosa of the human gastrointestinal tract is also impervious to bephenium, as it is to acetylcholine, presumably because these two compounds possess a quaternary nitrogen, i.e., a central nitrogen attached to four methyl groups. The poor absorption explains the low toxicity of this anthelmintic.

REFERENCES

1. Anderson JS, Meadow PM, Haskin MA, et al: Biosynthesis of the peptidoglycan of bacterial cell walls. I. Utilization of uridine diphosphate acetylmuramyl pentapeptide and uridine diphosphate acetylglucosamine for peptidoglycan synthesis by particulate enzymes from *Staphylococcus aureus* and *Micrococcus lysodeikticus*. Arch Biochem 116:487–515, 1966.
2. Appleyard G: Chemotherapy of viral infections. Br Med Bull 23:114–118, 1967.
3. Bueding E: Some biochemical effects of anthelmintic drugs. Biochem Pharmacol 18:1541–1547, 1969.
4. Bueding E, Fisher J: Biochemical effects of niridazole on *Schistosoma mansoni*. Molec Pharmacol 6:532–539, 1970.
5. Craven GR, Gavin R, Fanning T: The transfer RNA binding site of the 30 S ribosome and the site of tetracycline inhibition. Sympos Quant Biol 34:129–137, 1969.
6. Davis BD: Streptomycin resistance and the study of ribosomal structure and function. N Engl J Med 283:1405–1407, 1970.
7. De Kloet, SR: Effects of 5-fluorouracil and 6-azauracil on the synthesis of ribonucleic acid and protein in *Saccharomyces carlsbergensis*. Biochem J 106:167–178, 1968.
8. Del Castillo J, De Mello WC, Morales T: Mechanism of the paralysing action of piperazine on ascaris muscle. Br J Pharmacol 22:463–477, 1964.
9. Feingold DS: Antimicrobial chemotherapeutic agents: the nature of their action and selective toxicity. N Engl J Med 269:957–964, 1963.
10. Few AV: Interaction of polymyxin E with bacterial and other lipids. Biochim Biophys Acta 16:137–145, 1955.
11. Greenwood D: Mucopeptide hydrolases and bacterial "persisters." Lancet 2:465–466, 1972.
12. Grollman AP: Structural basis for inhibition of protein synthesis by emetine and cycloheximide based on an analogy between ipecac alkaloids and glutarimide antibiotics. Proc Nat Acad Sci USA 56:1867–1874, 1966.
13. Hahn FE, O'Brien RL, Ciak J, et al: Studies on modes of action of chloroquine, quinacrine, and quinine and on chloroquine resistance. Milit Med 131:Suppl:1071–1089, 1966.
14. Hitchings GH: Species differences among dihydrofolate reductases as a basis for chemotherapy. Postgrad Med J 45:Suppl:7–10, 1969.
15. Kaplan AS, Ben-Porat T: Differential incorporation of iododeoxyuridine into the DNA of pseudorabies virus-infected and noninfected cells. Virology 31:734–736, 1967.

16. Kinsky SC: Nystatin binding by protoplasts and a particulate fraction of *Neurospora crassa*, and a basis for the selective toxicity of polyene antifungal antibiotics. Proc Nat Acad Sci USA *48*.1049–1056, 1962.

17. Luzzato L, Apirion D, Schlessinger D: Mechanism of action of streptomycin in *E. coli:* interruption of the ribosome cycle at the initiation of protein synthesis. Proc Nat Acad Sci USA *60*:873–880, 1968.

18. Mao JC, Robishaw EE: Erythromycin, a peptidyl-transferase effector. Biochemistry *11*:4864–4872, 1972.

19. Neuhaus FC, Lynch JL: The enzymatic synthesis of D-alanyl-D-alanine. 3. On the inhibition of D-alanyl-D-alanine synthetase by the antibiotic D-cycloserine. Biochemistry (Wash) *3*:471–480, 1964.

20. Newton BA: The properties and mode of action of the polymyxins. Bacteriol Rev *20*: 14–27, 1956.

21. Ozaki M, Mizushima S, Nomura M: Identification and functional characterization of the protein controlled by the streptomycin-resistant locus in *E. coli.* Nature (London) *222*:333–339, 1969.

22. Pongs O, Bald R, Erdmann VA: Identification of chloramphenicol-binding protein in *Escherichia coli* ribosomes by affinity labeling. Proc Nat Acad Sci USA *70*:2229–2233, 1973.

23. Saz HJ: Comparative energy metabolisms of some parasitic helminths. J Parasitol *56*: 634–642, 1970.

24. Saz HJ, Bueding E: Relationships between anthelmintic effects and biochemical and physiological mechanisms. Pharmacol Rev *18*:871–894, 1966.

25. Siewert G, Strominger JL: Bacitracin: an inhibitor of the dephosphorylation of lipid pyrophosphate, an intermediate in biosynthesis of the peptidoglycan of bacterial cell walls. Proc Nat Acad Sci USA *57*:767–773, 1967.

26. Tipper DJ, Strominger JL: Mechanism of action of penicillins: a proposal based on their structural similarity to acyl-D-alanyl-D-alanine. Proc Nat Acad Sci USA *54*:1133–1141, 1965.

27. Van den Bossche H: Biochemical effects of the anthelmintic drug mebendazole. *In* Comparative Biochemistry of Parasites. Edited by Van den Bossche, H. New York, Academic Press, 1972, pp. 139–157.

28. Wehrli W, Staehelin M: Actions of the rifamycins. Bacteriol Rev *35*:290–309, 1971.

CHAPTER 3

MICROBIAL SUSCEPTIBILITY TO DRUGS

The antimicrobial activity of a drug is generally expressed as its minimum inhibitory concentration in nutrient broth or agar. The test conditions would seem far removed from those in infected tissues or body fluids, but there is a remarkable correlation between successful treatment of the patient and inhibitory concentrations in the laboratory.

Microbial inhibition is measured either by serial dilution or by diffusion of antibiotics.[41] In the dilution tests the antibiotic is diluted serially in broth or agar, and results are expressed as the lowest concentration that inhibits growth of a standard bacterial inoculum at 37°C. Three diffusion tests are used: the disk test, the filter strip, and the gradient plate. In the disk test, antibiotics are incorporated into filter paper disks, and the minimum inhibitory concentration is calculated indirectly from the diameter of the inhibitory zone[5, 17] (Fig. 3–1). Long filter paper strips can be used instead of disks. The strips have the advantage of measuring inhibitory concentrations against multiple strains of bacteria that are streaked perpendicularly to the strip.

The gradient plate is prepared by pouring agar with a given concentration of antibiotic in square Petri dishes that are tilted so that the agar solidifies on a slant. The plate is then placed on a flat surface and an equal volume of agar without antibiotic is poured over the slanted agar to provide a horizontal layer, as shown in Figure 3–2. The antibiotic diffuses into the upper layer to give a perfect linear gradient ranging from zero to the concentration present in the original layer. Multiple strains can be streaked on the agar surface along the gradient. The minimum inhibitory concentration is directly related to the distance bacterial growth extends from the zero end of the gradient.

The gradient plate method is the best method for laboratories that need to perform sensitivity on many strains because multiple organisms can

38

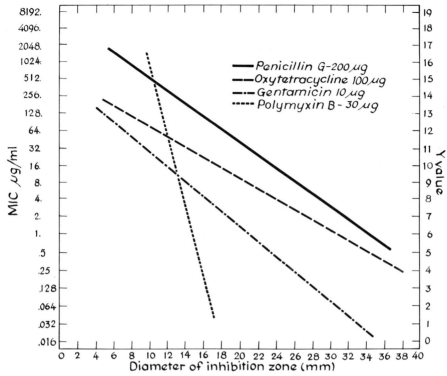

Figure 3–1. Determination of antibiotic sensitivity by disk method is based on correlation between zone diameter and minimum inhibitory concentration. Regression lines for minimum inhibitory concentrations and inhibitory zone diameter are shown for penicillin G (200 μg), oxytetracycline (100 μg), gentamicin (10 μg), and polymyxin B sulfate (30 μg). (From Stamey TA: Urinary Infections. Baltimore, The Williams & Wilkins Co., 1972, p. 45.)

be examined on one plate and there is little room for error.[7] The disk test is the most widely used (despite a number of disadvantages) because it lends itself to commercial distribution and has been publicized. The most serious problem encountered with the disk method is the occasional failure to detect strains of staphylococci that are resistant to penicillin. These resistant staphylococci are easily recognized by tests for penicillinase. The simplest is a rapid capillary tube assay that should be carried out routinely in all laboratories.[44] It is based on the change in pH that occurs when staphylococcal penicillinase hydrolyzes penicillin to penicilloic acid.

The values given below for antibiotic sensitivity are derived from either dilution methods or the gradient plate and are a composite of results from our laboratory and several other representative laboratories.

THE COCCI

With the exception of certain staphylococci, gonococci,[11, 42] and enterococci, cocci remain exquisitely sensitive to penicillin G (benzylpenicil-

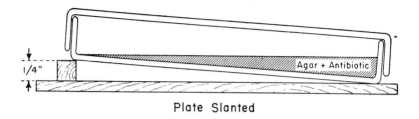

Plate Slanted

Plate Level

Figure 3-2. Diagram of procedures used for preparing gradient plates. The extreme right end of the completed plate (bottom) is where the gradient begins; there is initially no dilution of antibiotic at this point. Halfway across the plate (arrows) there is a twofold dilution of antibiotic. At the extreme left there is virtually no antibiotic and its concentration is zero. Thus a uniform linear gradient is formed by the vertical diffusion of antibiotic. (From Braude AI, Banister J, Wright N: Use of the gradient plate for routine clinical determinations of bacterial sensitivities to antibiotics. Antibiot Annu p. 1134, 1954–1955.)

lin). Pneumococci, hemolytic streptococci, meningococci, anaerobic streptococci, and *Streptococcus viridans* are usually inhibited by less than 0.1 microgram (μg) per ml and frequently by as little as 0.01 μg/ml[18, 34, 46] (Table 3–1). Gonococci and staphylococci are no longer uniformly sensitive to penicillin. Staphylococci that produce penicillinase cannot be treated with benzylpenicillin at any dosage. The number of staphylococci that produce penicillinase varies among hospitals. At the University Hospital in San Diego 80 per cent do so. Before 1960, 95 per cent of gonococci were sensitive to 0.1 μg/ml benzylpenicillin, but now less than half are inhibited by this concentration, and 1.0 μg/ml is necessary to inhibit 95 per cent of gonococcal strains in many communities.[32]

In contrast to those gonococci and staphylococci which have lost initial sensitivity, enterococci have always been relatively resistant to penicillin G. Enterococci generally grow readily in 1.0 μg/ml and usually require 3 to 6 μg/ml for inhibition.[18]

Modification of penicillin G to acid-resistant or penicillinase-resistant compounds causes loss in antibacterial power. In penicillin V and ampicillin the loss of activity against most cocci is usually slight; in fact, ampicillin is more active than penicillin G against the enterococci. *Neisseria* show the biggest differences in sensitivity between penicillin V and G, with the meningococcus and penicillin-sensitive gonococci requiring concentrations of penicillin V four times greater than those of penicillin G for inhibition.

The penicillinase-resistant penicillins show greater loss of activity

TABLE 3-1. Usual Minimum Inhibitory Concentrations (μg/ml) of Penicillin Derivatives Against Cocci

	BENZYL-PENICILLIN	PHENOXYMETHYL-PENICILLIN	AMPICILLIN*	METHICILLIN	OXACILLIN	DICLOXACILLIN	NAFCILLIN
Pneumococcus	0.01	0.03	0.02	—	0.5	0.15	0.04
Group A streptococcus	0.005	0.015	0.02	0.2	0.02	0.05	0.02
Staphylococcus aureus (penicillinase-negative)	0.03	0.03	0.05	1.0	0.30	0.15	0.40
S. aureus (penicillinase producer)	R	R	R	1.0	0.40	0.10	0.50
Streptococcus fecalis	3.6	3.2	1.6	>25.0	>25.0	—	25.0
Streptococcus viridans	0.01	—	0.1	0.1	—	—	—
Gonococcus	0.01–3.0	0.03–>3.0	0.3	—	—	—	—
Meningococcus	0.03	0.25	0.05	6.0	—	6.0	6.0
Peptostreptococcus	0.2	—	0.2	—	0.6	2.0	—

* The activity of amoxicillin is very similar to that of ampicillin, except for *Streptococcus fecalis*. Amoxicillin inhibits most strains of *S. fecalis* at 0.6 μg/ml.

R = Resistant at all concentrations.

— = Inadequate data.

TABLE 3–2. *Usual Minimum Inhibitory Concentrations (µg/ml) of Cephalosporin Antibiotics Against Cocci*[29, 47]

	CEPHALOTHIN	CEPHALEXIN	CEFAZOLIN
Pneumococcus	0.4	3.1	0.1
Group A streptococcus	0.1	1.0	0.2
Staphylococcus aureus	0.6	6.0	0.6
Staphylococcus epidermidis	0.6	—	1.0
Streptococcus fecalis	50.0	50.0	50.0
Streptococcus viridans	—	6.25	0.3
Gonococcus	4.0	6.0	4.0
Meningococcus	1.6	100.0	—

— = Inadequate data.

against penicillin-sensitive cocci. Methicillin is 35 to 40 times less active than penicillin G against streptococci and penicillinase-negative staphylococci. Cloxacillin, oxacillin, and dicloxacillin are approximately 8 to 12 times less active than penicillin G against pneumococci, various streptococci, and penicillinase-negative staphylococci.[22, 58] The same, except for a little more activity against the pneumococcus, is true for nafcillin. All four inhibit penicillinase-producing staphylococci in a range of 0.15 to 1 µg/ml.

The related group of penicillinase-resistant antibiotics, the cephalosporins, are also less active than penicillin against all cocci (Table 3–2). Cephaloridine approaches benzylpenicillin in potency *in vitro* against the pneumococcus and group A streptococcus but otherwise the cephalosporins are considerably less active against cocci than is benzylpenicillin.[25] The cephalosporins are so inactive against the enterococcus and meningococcus that they are virtually useless in infections with those organisms.[6, 47]

Tetracyclines are losing some of their potency against cocci.[18, 34] In all species of cocci, strains have appeared that are too resistant for treatment with this group of antibiotics. Resistance to tetracyclines has been most marked among the enterococci, but many staphylococci have also developed resistance beyond the limits of clinical efficacy. In certain hospitals as many as 50 per cent of staphylococci show such resistance while staphylococci from patients in outpatient clinics remain sensitive. So much resistance has developed among strains of pneumococci (5 to 23 per cent)

TABLE 3–3. *Usual Minimum Inhibitory Concentrations (µg/ml) of Tetracyclines Against Sensitive Strains of Cocci*

	TETRACYCLINE	DOXYCYCLINE	MINOCYCLINE
Staphylococcus aureus	0.3	0.8	0.8
Group A streptococcus	0.3	0.2	0.2
Pneumococcus	0.3	0.1	0.1
Peptostreptococcus	1.6	0.8	0.8
Gonococcus	0.8	0.8	0.8
Meningococcus	0.8	0.8	0.8

and group A streptococci (20 to 40 per cent)[34] that tetracyclines cannot be relied on for the treatment of pneumonia or sore throat unless sensitivity tests establish their susceptibility. Among anaerobic gram-positive cocci, tetracycline resistance is a lesser problem. In contrast to the aerobic gram-positive cocci, over 90 per cent of *Neisseria* remain sensitive to the tetracyclines, which can cure most cases of gonorrhea. One tetracycline, minocycline, has also been somewhat effective in treating pharyngeal carriers of meningococci.[21] The *in vitro* susceptibility of sensitive strains of cocci to the tetracyclines is shown in Table 3–3.

Certain tetracycline analogues seem to be more active *in vitro* against cocci that are resistant to other tetracyclines.[57] Minocycline is the best example of this phenomenon since it inhibits in low concentrations staphylococci, group A streptococci, and enterococci that are resistant to tetracycline.

Lincomycin and clindamycin inhibit most of the gram-positive cocci, but not the *Neisseria*. Clindamycin is 4 to 16 times more active than lincomycin against staphylococci, and the minimum inhibitory concentration (MIC) against hemolytic streptococci (groups A, B, and C), pneumococci, and *Streptococcus viridans* is less than 0.05 μg/ml.[12] Among gram-positive cocci, only enterococci are resistant. Anaerobic cocci are almost all sensitive to 1.0 μg/ml or less of clindamycin.

The spectrum of erythromycin resembles that of lincomycin and clindamycin except for the *Neisseria*.[12, 20] Most strains of gonococci and meningococci are inhibited by 1.0 μg/ml of erythromycin.[46] The pyogenic streptococci and pneumococci are inhibited by 0.04 μg/ml, and sensitive staphylococci by 0.4 μg/ml. Staphylococci sometimes become resistant to erythromycin, especially in the hospital, and may show cross resistance to lincomycin. Strains of group A streptococci[48] and pneumococci are rarely resistant, but in some large hospitals over half the strains of enterococci are resistant to erythromycin.[60] Other enterococci range in sensitivity from 0.1 to 1.5 μg/ml erythromycin. Most anaerobic streptococci also fall in this range of sensitivity.[33]

The cocci do not show the exquisite sensitivity to chloramphenicol often found with other antibiotics, but most cocci are inhibited by 1 to 4 μg/ml and acquired resistance is unusual. The average pneumococcus or group A streptococcus, for example, is inhibited by 3.0 μg/ml of chloramphenicol. Meningococci tend to be more sensitive, with the average strain inhibited by 1.0 μg/ml. Staphylococci, anaerobic cocci, enterococci, gonococci, and *Streptococcus viridans* are generally sensitive to 4 μg/ml or less.[18, 46]

The aminoglycosides are less active against cocci than other antibiotics that interfere with protein synthesis. Streptococci and pneumococci are naturally resistant, and the *Neisseria* generally show only marginal sensitivity. The staphylococci are an exception, because kanamycin and gentamicin are both highly active against them, and some strains are sensitive to streptomycin.[52] Staphylococci range in sensitivity to gentamicin from 0.1 to 1.0 μg/ml, and to kanamycin from 0.4 to 4.0 μg/ml. Spectinomycin is the only amino-glycoside with enough activity against the gonococcus to warrant its use for the routine treatment of gonorrhea. Gonococci range in sensitivity from 6.2 to 25 μg/ml.[24]

One of the most active antibiotics against cocci is rifampin. The MIC for group A streptococci, staphylococci, and pneumococci is 0.02 μg/ml or less, while meningococci are inhibited by 0.2 μg/ml, gonococci by 0.5 μg/ml, and anaerobic streptococci by 1.6 μg/ml.[28, 49] Only enterococci have too much innate resistance for clinical effectiveness of the drug. Acquired resistance to rifampin among staphylococci and other cocci occurs readily and limits its usefulness.

Only one other antibiotic, vancomycin, deserves brief mention for its use against cocci. Its main value is for enterococcal endocarditis in patients with severe penicillin allergy.[19] The MIC for vancomycin against enterococci is 0.3 to 3.0 μg/ml.

Most other antimicrobials have little place in the treatment of coccal infections. The polymyxins are inactive against cocci, and antimicrobials other than antibiotics are of such limited value that they need not be discussed here. An exception is trimethoprim, whose antimicrobial spectrum is described later.

THE BACILLI

Penicillin G is highly effective against all gram-positive bacilli and many gram-negative bacilli. Most enteric bacilli are relatively resistant but the penicillin derivatives, ampicillin and carbenicillin, usually inhibit these gram-negative rods in concentrations that can be reached in infected body fluids. The gram-positive rods, *Listeria monocytogenes, Actinomyces israelii,* the clostridia, *Erysipelothrix rhusiopathiae, Bacillus anthracis,* and

TABLE 3-4.   *Usual Minimum Inhibitory Concentrations (μg/ml) of Sensitive Bacilli to Benzylpenicillin*

Gram-positive rods	
Listeria monocytogenes	0.2
Actinomyces israelii	0.06
Clostridium perfringens	0.16
Bacillus anthracis	0.02
Corynebacterium diphtheriae	0.08
Erysipelothrix rhusiopathiae	0.03
Bordetella pertussis	0.5
Gram-negative rods	
Hemophilus influenzae	0.8
Pasteurella multocida	0.4
Streptobacillus moniliformis	0.01
Bacteroides oralis	1.6
Bacteroides melaninogenicus	1.0
Fusobacterium nucleatum	0.8

Corynebacterium diphtheriae, are all very sensitive to penicillin, and most are inhibited by less than 0.1 μg/ml. Certain important gram-negative rods such as *Hemophilus influenzae, Pasteurella multocida, Streptobacillus monilifor-mis,* and most *Bacteroides* other than *Bacteroides fragilis* are also sensitive to penicillin in a range of 0.5 to 2.0 μg/ml (Table 3–4). Despite impressions to the contrary, ampicillin is not superior to penicillin G against *H. influenzae.* Most careful studies in the United States have shown that the MIC of both antibiotics against *H. influenzae* ranges from 0.2 to 1.6 μg/ml, with a median near 0.8 μg/ml.[35, 46] A few strains have developed resistance, but since this is mediated by a β-lactamase, both drugs are ineffective against them.

Enteric bacilli are considerably less sensitive to penicillin G than the rods listed in Table 3–4.[18, 47, 56] Table 3–5 shows the greater susceptibility of these organisms to ampicillin and carbenicillin. Ampicillin inhibits sensitive strains of *Proteus mirabilis* and *E. coli* at a concentration of 3.0 μg/ml or less, and salmonellae at 6 μg/ml. Carbenicillin is active in a range achieved clinically against all gram-negative bacilli listed except for certain strains of *Serratia.*[10, 53]

The cephalosporins differ from the penicillins in the poor activity of the former against *H. influenzae* (Table 3–6). Another notable difference is the greater activity of cephalothin and cefazolin against *Klebsiella pneumoniae* than that shown by ampicillin and penicillin G. *Enterobacter aerogenes, Serratia,* indole + *Proteus,* and *Pseudomonas* are resistant to the cephalosporins.[15]

Erythromycin, lincomycin, and clindamycin are effective *in vitro* against *Bacteroides*[33] and the gram-positive rods, but not against enteric gram-negative bacilli. Erythromycin also shows activity against *H. influenzae* and *B. pertussis,* but lincomycin does not. Table 3–7 compares the activities of these three antibiotics against bacilli.

All the rods, both gram-positive and gram-negative, were initially sensitive to the tetracyclines and chloramphenicol, but some resistance has developed among the enteric bacilli. Table 3–8 shows that *Pseudomonas*

TABLE 3–5. *Comparison of Usual Minimum Inhibitory Concentrations (μg/ml) of Penicillin G, Ampicillin, and Carbenicillin for Enteric Gram-Negative Rods*

	BENZYLPENICILLIN	AMPICILLIN*	CARBENICILLIN
E. coli	100.0	3.0	12.0
P. mirabilis	50.0	3.0	1.6
K. pneumoniae	>100.0	25.0–400.0	>200.0
Enterobacter	>500.0	20.0–250.0	6.0
S. marcescens	>500.0	40.0–100.0	12.0–400.0
P. aeruginosa	>500.0	>200.0	50.0–100.0
Proteus vulgaris	>100.0	3.0–100.0	2.0–25.0
Other indole + *Proteus*	>100.0	3.0–50.0	1.0–12.0
Salmonella species	12.0	6.0	12.0
Pseudomonas pseudomallei	25.0	10.0	>100.0

* Amoxicillin activity against gram-negative rods is very similar to that of ampicillin except that amoxicillin is approximately four times as active against *Salmonella* strains.[38]

TABLE 3–6. *Usual Minimum Inhibitory Concentrations (µg/ml) of Cephalosporins for Pathogenic Bacilli*

	CEFAZOLIN	CEPHALOTHIN	CEPHALEXIN
Gram-positive rods			
Listeria monocytogenes	—	2.0	64.0
Actinomyces israelii	—	0.1	—
Clostridium perfringens	—	0.6	1.2
Bacillus anthracis	—	0.6	2.0
Gram-negative rods			
Hemophilus influenzae	25.0	6.0–10.0	6.0–20.0
Pasteurella multocida	—	0.6	2.0
Bacteroides fragilis	>200.0	25.0	25.0
Bacteroides oralis	—	0.1	—
Bacteroides melaninogenicus	—	0.2–6.0	—
Fusobacterium necrophorum	2.0	1.0	—
E. coli	0.8	6.0	12.0
P. mirabilis	3.0	6.0	20.0
K. pneumoniae	3.0	6.0	20.0
E. aerogenes	6.0–400.0	50.0->400.0	>100.0
S. marcescens	>400.0	> 100.0	>100.0
P. aeruginosa	>400.0	> 400.0	>100.0
Indole + *Proteus*	200.0	100.0–400.0	>100.0
Salmonella spp.	1.0	2.0	4.0
Shigella spp.	1.0	8.0	12.0
Pseudomonas pseudomallei	—	>1000.0	—

— = Inadequate data.

aeruginosa, Yersinia enterocolitica, indole + *Proteus*, and most *Serratia* are beyond the reach clinically of chloramphenicol and tetracycline.

The aminoglycosides differ from other antibiotics in the weakness of their inhibitory action against anaerobes[33] but show potent *in vitro* activity against nearly all other bacilli. The usual MIC of streptomycin, kanamycin, and gentamicin against aerobic gram-negative bacilli is given in Table 3–9. Two MIC values are given for a number of enteric bacteria because of differences in

TABLE 3–7. *Usual Minimum Inhibitory Concentrations (µg/ml) of Erythromycin, Lincomycin, and Clindamycin Against Susceptible Bacilli*

	ERYTHROMYCIN	LINCOMYCIN	CLINDAMYCIN
A. israelii	0.12	0.25	—
L. monocytogenes	2.0	—	—
C. diphtheriae	1.6	—	—
C. perfringens	1.5	2.0	0.8
B. anthracis	0.6	6.0	—
H. influenzae	3.0	20.0	6.0
P. multocida	3.1	—	—
B. fragilis	2.0	2.0	0.2
B. oralis	0.1	0.1	0.1
B. melaninogenicus	0.4	0.1	0.01
F. nucleatum	1.6	3.1	0.4

— = Inadequate data.

TABLE 3–8. *Usual Minimum Inhibitory Concentrations (μg/ml) of Gram-Positive and Gram-Negative Rods by Chloramphenicol and Tetracycline*

	CHLORAMPHENICOL	TETRACYCLINE
A. israelii	3.0	3.0
L. monocytogenes	5.0	1.0
C. diphtheriae	0.5	0.3–1.0
C. perfringens	3.0	3.0
B. anthracis	1.5	4.0
H. influenzae	2.0	2.0
B. pertussis	2.0	2.0
P. multocida	1.5	3.0
B. fragilis	6.0	1.0–25.0
B. oralis	1.5	0.5
B. melaninogenicus	1.5	1.0
F. nucleatum	3.1	6.2
E. coli	6.0–12.0	6.0–50.0
E. aerogenes	20.0	50.0–>100.0
K. pneumoniae	10.0	50.0–>100.0
S. marcescens	25.0	100.0
P. mirabilis	6.0–12.0	50.0–100.0
Indole + Proteus	50.0	25.0
P. aeruginosa	>100.0	>100.0
Y. enterocolitica[64]	3.0	6.0
B. abortus[63]	3.0	1.0
P. pseudomallei[16]	6.4	1.6
Salmonella spp.	2.0	1.0
Shigella spp.	2.0	8.0
Vibrio cholerae[30]	1.25	1.05

TABLE 3–9. *Sensitivity in vitro of Gram-Negative Bacilli to Aminoglycosides*

	USUAL MINIMUM INHIBITORY CONCENTRATIONS (μg/ml)		
	Streptomycin	Kanamycin	Gentamicin
H. influenzae	8.0	4.0	2.0
B. pertussis	4.0	2.0	1.0
P. multocida	25.0	—	—
E. coli	4.0–25.0	3.0	2.0
E. aerogenes	4.0–25.0	2.0–10.0	0.5–2.0
K. pneumoniae	6.0–100.0	2.0–10.0	1.0–4.0
S. marcescens	>100.0	10.0	4.0
P. mirabilis	6.0–>100.0	2.0–>100.0	0.3–5.0
Indole + Proteus	6.0–>100.0	2.0–>100.0	2.0
P. aeruginosa	50.0	>100.0	1.0–4.0
P. pseudomallei	>200.0	25.6	50.0
Y. enterocolitica[64]	6.0–>100.0	6.0	—
B. abortus[63]	2.0	1.5	0.3
Salmonella spp.	4.0–16.0	3.0	0.8
Shigella spp.	3.0–10.0	5.0	2.0
Francisella tularensis[3]	0.4	—	—
Vibrio cholerae	20.0	—	—

— = Inadequate data.

TABLE 3–10.   *Sensitivity of Gram-Negative Bacilli to Rifampin*

ORGANISM	USUAL MINIMUM INHIBITORY CONCENTRATIONS (μg/ml)
E. coli	2.5–10.0
P. mirabilis	1.0
Indole + Proteus	3.0
P. aeruginosa	10.0
Salmonella spp.	7.5
Shigella spp.	2.5
K. pneumoniae	10.0
P. pseudomallei	50.0
H. influenzae	0.2–0.8

susceptibility between "street" and "hospital" strains and because of variations from one community or hospital to another. The *in vitro* sensitivities of *Salmonella* and *Brucella* are misleading because streptomycin and kanamycin are not effective in treating brucellosis or *Salmonella* infections.

The polymyxins—polymyxin B and colistin methane sulfonate—are also impotent against the anaerobes, as well as the gram-negative bacilli, *Proteus*, *Serratia*, *Brucella*, and *P. pseudomallei*. Most strains of *E. coli*, *K. pneumoniae*, and *P. aeruginosa* are inhibited by 2.5 μg/ml or less of either drug. *Salmonella*, *Shigella*, and *H. influenzae* are even more sensitive (0.2 to 0.4 μg/ml), but the polymyxins are seldom used to treat infections by these three groups of organisms.

Rifampin is effective to some degree against all the enteric rods and *H. influenzae* [2, 26, 49] (Table 3–10).

Among the sulfonamides, sulfadiazine and sulfisoxazole will inhibit most enteric bacilli in concentrations of 8 to 64 μg/ml in the absence of acquired resistance. Of the gram-negative rods, *P. aeruginosa* is most likely to be innately resistant to these concentrations. Acquired resistance to sulfonamides is so common among all bacteria, however, that sensitivity tests are usually needed to predict results.

Many gram-negative bacilli are also susceptible to nalidixic acid in concentrations of 20 to 50 μg/ml. *Klebsiella*, *E. coli*, *P. mirabilis*, and indole + *Proteus* organisms are often sensitive, while *P. aeruginosa* is uniformly resistant. Resistance tends to develop so rapidly, however, that it can appear overnight during treatment with nalidixic acid.[43, 54]

Metronidazole, a drug with interesting potential activity in anaerobic infections, can inhibit *B. fragilis* and other species of the family Bacteroidaceae. Concentrations of 3.1 μg/ml inhibit most *B. fragilis*.[59]

OTHER PATHOGENIC MICROORGANISMS

Mycobacteria and Nocardia

Mycobacteria show a different pattern of drug susceptibility than that of most bacteria (Table 3–11). Among antibiotics in general use in various

TABLE 3-11. *Drug Sensitivity of Mycobacteria*

USUAL MINIMUM INHIBITORY CONCENTRATIONS (μg/ml)

	M. tuberculosis var. hominis	M. kansasii	M. marinum	M. intracellulare	M. fortuitum
Isoniazide	0.2	>25.0	>25.0	>25.0	>25.0
Rifampin	0.1	0.1–0.5	0.6	10.0	>20.0
Ethambutol	1.0	5.0	—	—	>20.0
Streptomycin	0.3–6.0	12.0–25.0	2.0–10.0	12.0–25.0	>100.0
Kanamycin	8.0	>5.0	5.0	—	—
Erythromycin	>32.0	1.0–2.0	—	32.0	>32.0
Tetracycline	10.0	—	—	—	—
PAS	1.0	>10.0	>2.0	—	>10.0
Pyrazinamide	18.0–20.0	>100.0	50.0	>100.0	—
Cycloserine	5.0–20.0	>50.0	50.0	—	>100.0
Gentamicin	3.0–6.0	3.0	—	3.0	25.0

— = Inadequate data.

bacterial infections, only the aminoglycosides and rifampin are active enough to warrant extensive use in tuberculosis and other mycobacterial infections.[28, 40] In fact, the most important antituberculosis drug, isoniazid, has no significant inhibitory effect on any other group of bacteria. The same is true of ethambutol and pyrazinamide. Despite its spectacular activity against human and bovine tubercle bacilli, isoniazid is inactive against most mycobacteria. Some other mycobacteria, especially *Mycobacterium kansasii*, are very sensitive to rifampin (but not rifamycin) and are moderately sensitive to streptomycin.[31] This organism is also sensitive *in vitro* to erythromycin. The major difference in susceptibility between the human and bovine tubercle bacillus is that *M. tuberculosis* var. *bovis* is resistant to pyrazinamide while *M. tuberculosis* var. *hominis* is sensitive. The slight sensitivity of the human tubercle bacillus to tetracycline has had some practical implications in combined drug therapy for preventing resistance to another antituberculous drug, but not for primary treatment.

Nocardia asteroides, the only important acid-fast bacillus other than the mycobacteria, is resistant to most antimycobacterial drugs. In general, strains of *Nocardia* show considerable variation in susceptibility to a given drug but are usually sensitive *in vitro* to the sulfonamides, tetracyclines, and cycloserine. The most consistently active antibiotic *in vitro* is minocycline, which inhibits 90 per cent of nocardial strains at a concentration of 3.1 μg/ml.[4] Erythromycin inhibits 40 per cent of strains at 0.8 μg/ml, but the others are resistant to >100 μg/ml. These *in vitro* results, based on standard testing methods, are probably not applicable to clinical therapy because the sulfonamides have been the most consistently successful drug for treating human nocardiosis even though *Nocardia* strains are highly resistant (>1600 μg/ml) to sulfonamides *in vitro* unless tiny inocula (<100 organisms) are used. Likewise, a number of patients have not responded to antibiotics that inhibited the infecting strain of *Nocardia* in low concentrations *in vitro*.

Mycoplasma

Mycoplasma pneumoniae, the cause of primary atypical pneumonia, is the only mycoplasma which has been proved to cause human infection, although T mycoplasma has been implicated in nongonococcal urethritis. Both organisms are resistant to drugs that affect the mucopeptide of bacteria because this structure is not present in mycoplasma. Their *in vitro* sensitivities are given in Table 3–12.[8, 39] Erythromycin and tetracycline are active against them, while lincomycin and clindamycin are ineffective.

Yeasts and Fungi

Amphotericin B, 5-fluorocytosine, nystatin, and griseofulvin are the major drugs given for treating fungus infections. Amphotericin B and 5-fluorocytosine are active against the fungi causing deep mycoses, and griseofulvin against dermatophytes. Nystatin is used only topically. The sulfonamides, clotrimazole, and hydroxystilbamidine have some antifungal

TABLE 3–12. In Vitro *Sensitivity of Mycoplasmas to Antibiotics*

	USUAL MINIMUM INHIBITORY CONCENTRATIONS (μg/ml)	
	M. pneumoniae	*T Mycoplasma*
Tetracycline	1.6	0.4
Erythromycin	0.025	1.6
Lincomycin	20.0	200.0
Chloramphenicol	12.0	1.6
Streptomycin	1.0	1.6
Polymyxin	—	500.0
Kanamycin	—	3.1
Gentamicin	—	6.2
Clindamycin	—	6.2–50.0

— = Inadequate data.

properties, but toxicity (clotrimazole, hydroxystilbamidine) or narrow spectrum (sulfonamides) greatly limits their use. Their activity against sensitive strains *in vitro* [1, 13, 14, 23, 27, 50, 51, 55, 61] is summarized in Table 3–13.

Griseofulvin inhibits virtually all dermatophytes at a concentration of less than 0.5 μg/ml. *Microsporum canis, M. gypseum, M. audouinii, Epidermophyton floccosum, Trichophyton mentagrophytes, T. rubrum, T. tonsurans, T. versicolor,* and all other clinically significant dermatophytes are susceptible in tube dilution tests to this concentration, or less, of griseofulvin.[45]

SYNERGISM

A few important drugs are more active in the presence of another. The second drug can potentiate by increasing permeability. Thus, the aminoglycosides are more active with penicillin, while rifampicin, 5-fluorocytosine, and tetracycline are potentiated against fungi by amphotericin B. By injuring the mucopeptide of the cell wall, penicillin facilitates entry

TABLE 3–13. *Usual Minimum Inhibitory Concentrations (μg/ml)*

	AMPHOTERICIN	5-FLUOROCYTOSINE	CLOTRIMAZOLE	NYSTATIN
Cryptococcus neoformans	0.4–3.0	0.5–4.0	1.6	1.5
Coccidioides immitis	0.5	>100.0	0.4	1.5
Aspergillus fumigatus	>40.0	50.0– > 100.0	1.6	3.0
Blastomyces dermatiditis	0.4–0.8	25.0	0.2	0.8
Candida albicans	2.0–4.0	0.5–500.0	4.0–16.0	3.0
Torulopsis glabrata	0.5–2.0	0.5–5.0	2.0–8.0	—
Histoplasma capsulatum	0.1–0.8	>100.0	3.0	1.5
Sporothrix schenckii	0.1–0.6	>100.0	—	12.0
Mucoraceae	0.03– > 2.5	>100.0	0.8	12.0

— = Inadequate data.

TABLE 3-14. *Synergism between Trimethoprim and Sulfamethoxazole*[9]

	USUAL MINIMUM INHIBITORY CONCENTRATIONS (μg/ml)			
	Sulfamethoxazole Alone	*Trimethoprim Alone*	*Sulfamethoxazole in Combination*	*Trimethoprim in Combination*
Streptococcus pyogenes	100.0	1.0	1.0	0.05
Pneumococcus	30.0	2.0	2.0	0.1
S. aureus	3.0	1.0	0.3	0.015
H. influenzae	10.0	1.0	0.3	0.015
K. pneumoniae	100.0	3.0	4.0	0.2
E. coli	3.0	0.3	1.0	0.05
Salmonella typhimurium	10.0	1.0	0.3	0.05
Shigella sonnei	>10.0	1.0	0.3	0.05
N. gonorrhoeae	5.0	18.3	4.0	2.3

so that more of the aminoglycoside can reach the ribosomes.[37, 65] Amphotericin B alters permeability by binding with sterols so that more 5-fluorocytosine can enter the cells and inhibit nucleic acid synthesis through its action on pyrimidine biosynthesis.[36] This idea is the basis for the combined treatment of cryptococcosis with amphotericin B plus 5-fluorocytosine, and of enterococcal endocarditis with streptomycin and penicillin. More than 50 μg/ml streptomycin and more than 100 μg/ml penicillin are required to kill most enterococci, but many of these are killed by 6.25 μg of streptomycin in the presence of 6.25 μg penicillin or less.[62] In other words, one-fourth or less of the minimum bactericidal concentration of each drug alone killed enterococci in combination. Similar synergism against enterococci occurs with penicillin plus kanamycin and with penicillin plus gentamicin.

A second drug can also potentiate by reinforcing the metabolic disturbance of the first. This approach is used for synergism between trimethoprim and sulfonamides, two drugs that block two sequential steps in folinic acid synthesis.[9] Maximum potentiation occurs when the two drugs are present in proportions corresponding to their respective MIC when acting singly. Trimethoprim is usually about 20 times more active than sulfamethoxazole, the sulfonamide with which it is usually combined. When the two drugs are mixed according to this ratio (20 sulf:1 trimethoprim),

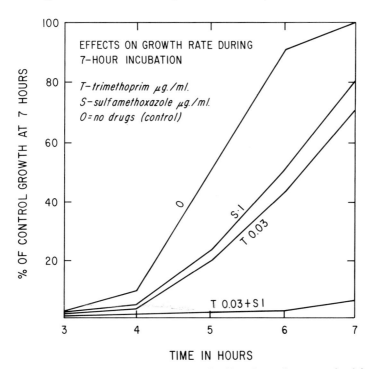

Figure 3–3. Synergism between trimethoprim and sulfamethoxazole on growth inhibition of *E. coli*. (Modified from Bushby SRM: Combined antibacterial action *in vitro* of trimethoprim and sulphonamides. Postgrad Med J 45:17, Nov 1969.)

they potentiate each other against many organisms, including streptococci, pneumococci, *S. aureus, H. influenzae, B. pertussis, K. pneumoniae, E. coli, Salmonella, Shigella, Proteus,* and gonococci. Examples are given in Table 3–14 and Figure 3–3, which give the minimum inhibitory concentrations of each drug when they are combined in a ratio of 1 part trimethoprim and 20 parts sulfamethoxazole.[9] The results show a potentiation of at least twentyfold for each drug against most organisms when used in combination.

REFERENCES

1. Artis D, Baum GL: In vitro susceptibility of 24 strains of *Histoplasma capsulatum* to amphotericin B. Antibiot Chemother *11*:373–376, 1961.
2. Atlas E, Turck M: Laboratory and clinical evaluation of rifampicin. Am J Med Sci *256*:47–54, 1968.
3. Avery FW, Barnett TB: Pulmonary tularemia. A report of five cases and consideration of pathogenesis and terminology. Am Rev Resp Dis *95*:584–591, 1967.
4. Bach MC, Sabath LD, Finland M: Susceptibility of *Nocardia asteroides* to 45 antimicrobial agents in vitro. Antimicrob Agents Chemother *3*:1–8, 1973.
5. Bauer AW, Kirby WM, Sherris JC, et al: Antibiotic susceptibility testing by a standardized single disk method. Am J Clin Pathol *45*:493–496, 1966.
6. Benner EJ: The cephalosporin antibiotics. Pediatr Clin North Am *15*:31–42, 1968.
7. Braude AI, Banister J, Wright N: Use of the gradient plate for routine clinical determinations of bacterial sensitivities to antibiotics. Antibiot Annu 1133–1140, 1954–1955.
8. Braun P, Klein JO, Kass EH: Susceptibility of genital mycoplasmas to antimicrobial agents. Appl Microbiol *19*:62–70, 1970.
9. Bushby RS: Combined antibacterial action in vitro of trimethoprim and sulphonamides. The in vitro nature of synergy. Postgrad Med J *45*:Suppl:10–18, 1969.
10. Butler K, English AR, Ray VA, et al: Carbenicillin: chemistry and mode of action. J Infect Dis *122*:Suppl:S1–8, 1970.
11. Cave VG, Hurdle ES, Catelli AR: Sensitivity of *Neisseria gonorrhoeae* to penicillin and other drugs. NY State J Med *70*:844–847, 1970.
12. Chadwick P: Bacteriological assessment of clindamycin, a new lincomycin derivative. J Med Microbiol *4*:529–534, 1971.
13. Drouhet E: Basic mechanisms of antifungal chemotherapy. Mod Treat *7*:539–564, 1970.
14. Drutz DJ, Spickard A, Rogers DE, et al: Treatment of disseminated mycotic infections. A new approach to amphotericin B therapy. Am J Med *45*:405–418, 1968.
15. Edmondson EB, Sanford JP: The Klebsiella-Enterobacter (Aerobacter)-Serratia group. A clinical and bacteriological evaluation. Medicine (Balt) *46*:323–340, 1967.
16. Eickhoff TC, Bennett JV, Hayes PS, et al: *Pseudomonas pseudomallei*: susceptibility to chemotherapeutic agents. J Infect Dis *121*:95–102, 1970.
17. Ericsson H, Hogman C, Wickman K: Paper disc method for determination of bacterial sensitivity to chemotherapeutic and antibiotic agents. Scand J Clin Lab Invest *6*:Suppl:21–36, 1954.
18. Finland M: Changing patterns of susceptibility of common bacterial pathogens to antimicrobial agents. Ann Intern Med *76*:1009–1036, 1972.
19. Friedberg CK, Rosen KM, Bienstock PA: Vancomycin therapy for enterococcal and *Streptococcus viridans* endocarditis. Successful treatment of six patients. Arch Intern Med (Chicago) *122*:134–140, 1968.
20. Griffith RS, Black HR: Erythromycin. Med Clin North Am *54*:1199–1215, 1970.
21. Guttler RB, Counts GW, Avent CK, et al: Effect of rifampin and minocycline on meningococcal carrier rates. J Infect Dis *24*:199–205, 1971.
22. Hammerstrom CF, Cox F, McHenry MC, et al: Clinical, laboratory, and pharmacological studies of dicloxacillin. Antimicrob Agents Chemother 69–74, 1966.
23. Hildick-Smith G: Antifungal antibiotics. Pediatr Clin North Am *15*:107–118, 1968.
24. Judson FN, Allaman J, Dans PE: Treatment of gonorrhea—Comparison of penicillin G procaine, doxycycline, spectinomycin, and ampicillin. JAMA *230*:705–708, 1974.

25. Kayser FH: In vitro activity of cephalosporin antibiotics against gram-positive bacteria. Postgrad Med J 47:Suppl:14–20, 1971.
26. Kunin CM, Brandt D, Wood H: Bacteriologic studies of rifampin, a new semisynthetic antibiotic. J Infect Dis 119:132–137, 1969.
27. Larsh HW, Hinton A, Silberg SL: The use of the tissue culture method in evaluating antifungal agents against systemic fungi. Antibiot Annu 988–991, 1957–1958.
28. Lester W: Rifampin: a semisynthetic derivative of rifamycin—a prototype for the future. Am Rev Microbiol 26:85–102, 1972.
29. Levison ME, Johnson WD, Thornhill TS, et al: Clinical and in vitro evaluation of cephalexin. A new orally administered cephalosporin antibiotic. JAMA 209:1331–1336, 1969.
30. Lindenbaum J, Greenough WB, Islam MR: Antibiotic therapy of cholera. Bull WHO 36:871–883, 1967.
31. Lorian V, Finland M: In vitro effect of rifampin on mycobacteria. Appl Microbiol 17:202–207, 1969.
32. Martin JE Jr, Lester A, Kellogg DS Jr, et al: In vitro susceptibility of Neisseria gonorrhoeae to nine antimicrobial agents. Appl Microbiol 18:21–23, 1969.
33. Martin WJ, Gardner M, Washington JA II: In vitro antimicrobial susceptibility of anaerobic bacteria isolated from clinical specimens. Antimicrob Agents Chemother 1:148–158, 1972.
34. Matsen JM, Blazevic DJ, Chapman SS: In vitro susceptibility patterns of beta-hemolytic streptococci. Antimicrob Agents Chemother 485–488, 1969.
35. McLinn SE, Nelson JD, Haltalin KC: Antimicrobial susceptibility of Hemophilus influenzae. Pediatrics 45:827–838, 1970.
36. Medoff G, Comfort M, Kobayashi GS: Synergistic action of amphotericin B and 5-fluorocytosine against yeast-like organisms. Proc Soc Exp Biol Med 138:571–574, 1971.
37. Moellering RC Jr, Wennersten C, Weinberg AN: Studies on antibiotic synergism against enterococci. I. Bacteriologic studies. J Lab Clin Med 77:821–828, 1971.
38. Neu H: Antimicrobial activity and human pharmacology of amoxicillin. J Infect Dis 129:Suppl:S123–131, 1974.
39. Niitu Y, Hasegawa S, Suetake T, et al: Resistance of Mycoplasma pneumoniae to erythromycin and other antibiotics. J Pediatr 76:438–443, 1970.
40. Raleigh JW: Rifampin in treatment of advanced pulmonary tuberculosis. Report of a VA cooperative pilot study. Am Rev Respir Dis 105:397–409, 1972.
41. Ribble JC: Laboratory assistance in the treatment of bacterial infections. Pediatr Clin North Am 18:115–124, 1971.
42. Ronald AR, Eby J, Sherris JC: Susceptibility of Neisseria gonorrhoeae to penicillin and tetracycline. Antimicrob Agents Chemother 431–434, 1968.
43. Ronald AR, Turck M, Petersdorf RG: A critical evaluation of nalidixic acid in urinary-tract infections. N Engl J Med 275:1081–1089, 1966.
44. Rosen IG, Jacobsen J, Rudderman R: Rapid capillary tube method for detecting penicillin resistance in Staphylococcus aureus. Appl Microbiol 23:649–650, 1972.
45. Roth FJ, Sallman B, Blank H: In vitro studies of the antifungal antibiotic griseofulvin. J Invest Dermatol 33:403–418, 1959.
46. Sabath LD, Stumpf LL, Wallace SJ, et al: Susceptibility of Diplococcus pneumoniae, Hemophilus influenzae, and Neisseria meningitidis to 23 antibiotics. Antimicrob Agents Chemother 53–56, 1970.
47. Sabath LD, Wilcox C, Garner C, et al: In vitro activity of cefazolin against recent clinical bacterial isolates. J Infect Dis 128:Suppl:S320–326, 1973.
48. Sanders E, Foster MT, Scott D: Group A beta-hemolytic streptococci resistant to erythromycin and lincomycin. N Engl J Med 278:538–540, 1968.
49. Sensi P, Maggi N, Füresz S, et al: Chemical modifications and biological properties of rifamycins. Antimicrob Agents Chemother 699–714, 1966.
50. Shadomy S: Further in vitro studies with 5-fluorocytosine. Infect Immunol 2:484–488, 1970.
51. Shadomy S, Kirchoff CB, Ingroff AE: In vitro activity of 5-fluorocytosine against Candida and Torulopsis species. Antimicrob Agents Chemother 3:9–14, 1973.
52. Simon HJ: Streptomycin, kanamycin, neomycin, and paromomycin. Pediatr Clin North Am 15:73–83, 1968.
53. Smith CB, Wilfert JN, Dans PE, et al: In-vitro activity of carbenicillin and results of treatment of infections due to Pseudomonas with carbenicillin singly and in combination with gentamicin. J Infect Dis 122:Suppl:S14–28, 1970.

54. Stamey TA, Nemoy NJ, Higgins M: The clinical use of nalidixic acid. A review and some observations. Invest Urol 6:582–592, 1969.
55. Steer PL, Marks MI, Klite PD, et al: 5-Fluorocytosine: an oral antifungal compound. A report on clinical and laboratory experience. Ann Intern Med 76:15–22, 1972.
56. Steigbigel NH, McCall CE, Reed CW, et al: Antibacterial action of "broad-spectrum" penicillins, cephalosporins and other antibiotics against gram-negative bacilli isolated from bacteremic patients. Ann NY Acad Sci 145:224–236, 1967.
57. Steigbigel NH, Reed CW, Finland M: Susceptibility of common pathogenic bacteria to seven tetracycline antibiotics in vitro. Am J Med Sci 255:179–195, 1968.
58. Sutherland R, Croydon EA, Rolinson GN: Flucloxacillin, a new isoxazolyl penicillin, compared with oxacillin, cloxacillin, and dicloxacillin. Br Med J 4:455, 1970.
59. Tally FP, Sutter VL, Finegold SM: Metronidazole versus anaerobes. In vitro data and initial clinical observations. Calif Med 117:22–26, 1972.
60. Toala P, McDonald A, Wilcox C, et al: Comparison of antibiotic susceptibility of group D streptococcus strains isolated at Boston City Hospital in 1953–54 and 1968–69. Antimicrob Agents Chemother 479–484, 1969.
61. Watson DC, Neame PB: In vitro activity of amphotericin B on strains of *Mucoraceae* pathogenic to man. J Lab Clin Med 56:251–257, 1960.
62. Wilkowske CJ, Facklam RR, Washington JA II, Geraci J: Antibiotic synergism: enhanced susceptibility of group D streptococci to certain antibiotic combinations. Antimicrob Agents Chemother 195–200, 1970.
63. Yow EM, Spink WW: Symposium on antibiotics; experimental studies on the action of streptomycin, aureomycin, and chloromycetin on brucella. J Clin Invest 28:871–885, 1949.
64. Zen-Yoji H, Maruyama T: The first successful isolations and identification of *Yersinia enterocolitica* from human cases in Japan. Jap J Microbiol 16:493–500, 1972.
65. Zimmermann RA, Moellering RC Jr, Weinberg AN: Mechanism of resistance to antibiotic synergism in enterococci. J Bacteriol 105:873–879, 1971.

CHAPTER 4

ACQUIRED RESISTANCE TO ANTIMICROBIAL DRUGS

Microbial resistance is acquired after a change in DNA. This change may occur by alteration in structure of chromosomal DNA or by acquisition of extrachromosomal DNA. The alteration of chromosomal DNA is called mutation, and the acquisition of extrachromosomal DNA is the result of genetic exchange. These changes lead to the formation of enzymes or other proteins that inactivate drugs or hinder access to their site of action.

MECHANISMS OF DRUG RESISTANCE

Genetic exchange is the more important cause of clinical drug resistance because it produces epidemic resistance to multiple drugs.[28] The extrachromosomal DNA responsible for such resistance can reproduce itself within the bacterial cell and then spread to other bacteria by transduction or by mating (conjugation).[21] Transduction is a type of gene transfer in which DNA from one bacterial cell is introduced into another bacterial cell by bacteriophage infection. The transmission of resistance from one bacterial cell to another is known as "infectious" drug resistance because sensitive bacteria become "infected" with resistance determinants. By this process, resistance to one or several antibiotics may spread from one bacterium to another during mating even in the absence of antibiotics. In other words, bacteria may become resistant to multiple drugs without ever having been exposed to them.

The genetic elements which control infectious drug resistance are a form of DNA known as plasmids. Plasmids are not part of the large circular bacterial chromosome but exist as small cyclic DNA molecules capable of reproducing themselves independently. The extrachromosomal resistance factors in gram-negative bacteria are called R factors.[28] R factors are composed of two kinds of genes: those that carry determinants for antibiotic resistance and those that promote transfer from one cell to another. The first are called resistance determinants (RD), and the second are resistance transfer factors (RTF). The R factor is transferred (during mating) via external hairlike appendages, the sex pili, from male (donor) bacteria to female recipients, which have no pili (Fig. 4–1). The number of RDs attached to RTFs determines the number of drugs to which the bacteria become resistant. One R factor may have as many as seven genes, each responsible for resistance to a different antibiotic. [6, 28] RTFs and RDs may reproduce themselves independently, and each may be present in the absence of the other. Bacteria containing only one of the two cannot transfer drug resistance, but can mate with a bacterium containing the other to produce cells with complete R factor. When a bacterium becomes infected with an R factor, the cell develops sex pili and becomes a donor cell. Donor competence, or the capacity to transfer resistance by conjugation, is greatest in bacteria that have recently acquired an R factor. The number of cells that are competent donors declines after a few generations as the capacity to produce sex pili is repressed.

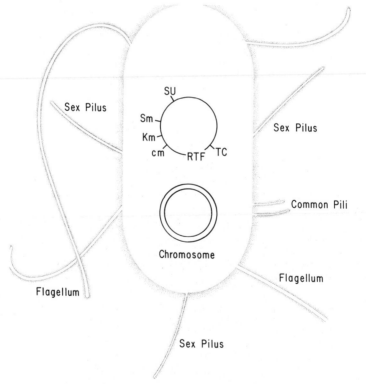

Figure 4–1. The genes carrying resistance determinants to antibiotics are carried outside the chromosome on R factors. The R factor is transferred during mating from male (donor) bacteria via the sex pili to female recipients which have no pili. The genes illustrated here determine resistance for chloramphenicol (cm), kanamycin (Km), streptomycin (Sm), sulfonamides (SU), and tetracycline (TC).

R factors are found mainly in intestinal bacteria, especially in *E. coli*, *Enterobacter aerogenes*, *K. pneumoniae*, *Salmonella*, *Shigella*, *Proteus*, and *Pseudomonas*. Since R factors can be transferred from one bacterial species to another, regardless of pathogenicity, they can be transferred from resistant *E. coli* to *Salmonella* or *Shigella* within the human bowel.[4] Bacteria containing R factors are a serious problem in the chemotherapy of such diseases as typhoid fever and bacillary dysentery because they retain virulence.

No single mechanism is responsible for resistance in bacteria carrying R factors. Penicillin and cephalosporin resistance, for example, is due to hydrolytic enzymes that open the β-lactam ring.[2, 8] Two general types of β-lactamases occur: one active mainly against penicillin and the other against both penicillin and cephalosporin. Penicillinase is situated on the cytoplasmic membrane and destroys the antibiotic as it permeates the cell wall. The other enzymes mediating R factor resistance are intracellular and not hydrolytic. They inactivate antibiotics by conjugating them with acetyl, phosphoryl, or adenyl groups. Chloramphenicol is inactivated by the enzyme chloramphenicol acetyltransferase in the presence of two intracellular metabolites, ATPase (adenosine triphosphatase) and acetyl CoA (coenzyme A).[22, 25, 26] Kanamycin can be inactivated by an acetyltransferase but is more often inactivated by the enzyme kanamycin-monophosphotransferase, which phosphorylates the drug in the presence of ATP.[22, 27] Streptomycin is inactivated by phosphorylation through the action of a streptomycin-phosphorylase, and by adenylation with streptomycin-adenyltransferase in the presence of ATP[30] (Fig. 4–2).

Transferable tetracycline resistance results from changes in the permeability of the bacterial cells to the drugs.[10] Tetracycline appears to leave the cell so rapidly that effective intracellular concentrations are not maintained. In other words, increased permeability allows the drug to flow out of the cell.[11] Sulfonamide resistance is also a result of a permeability change, but the mechanism has not been studied enough to determine if the process is like that for tetracycline or if it involves impermeability.

In staphylococci the plasmids controlling drug resistance are transferred only by transduction and not by mating. Resistance to penicillin is due to the production of a β-lactamase by penicillinase plasmids. These plasmids may also be the site of genetic markers for erythromycin, but resistance to streptomycin, tetracycline, and chloramphenicol is located on different plasmids.[21]

In contrast to infectious drug resistance, resistance after mutation involves chromosomal genes. Spontaneous mutation to drug resistance is infrequent, generally occurring in only 1 of 10,000,000 to 1,000,000,000,000 bacterial cells. The resistant mutants are difficult to detect unless the drug is present as a selective agent to suppress the overwhelming number of nonmutated cells and allow multiplication of those which are resistant. Multiplication of resistant organisms during antibiotic therapy usually occurs on mucous membranes, in urine, or in lung cavities where there are no immune mechanisms to check the growth of the or-

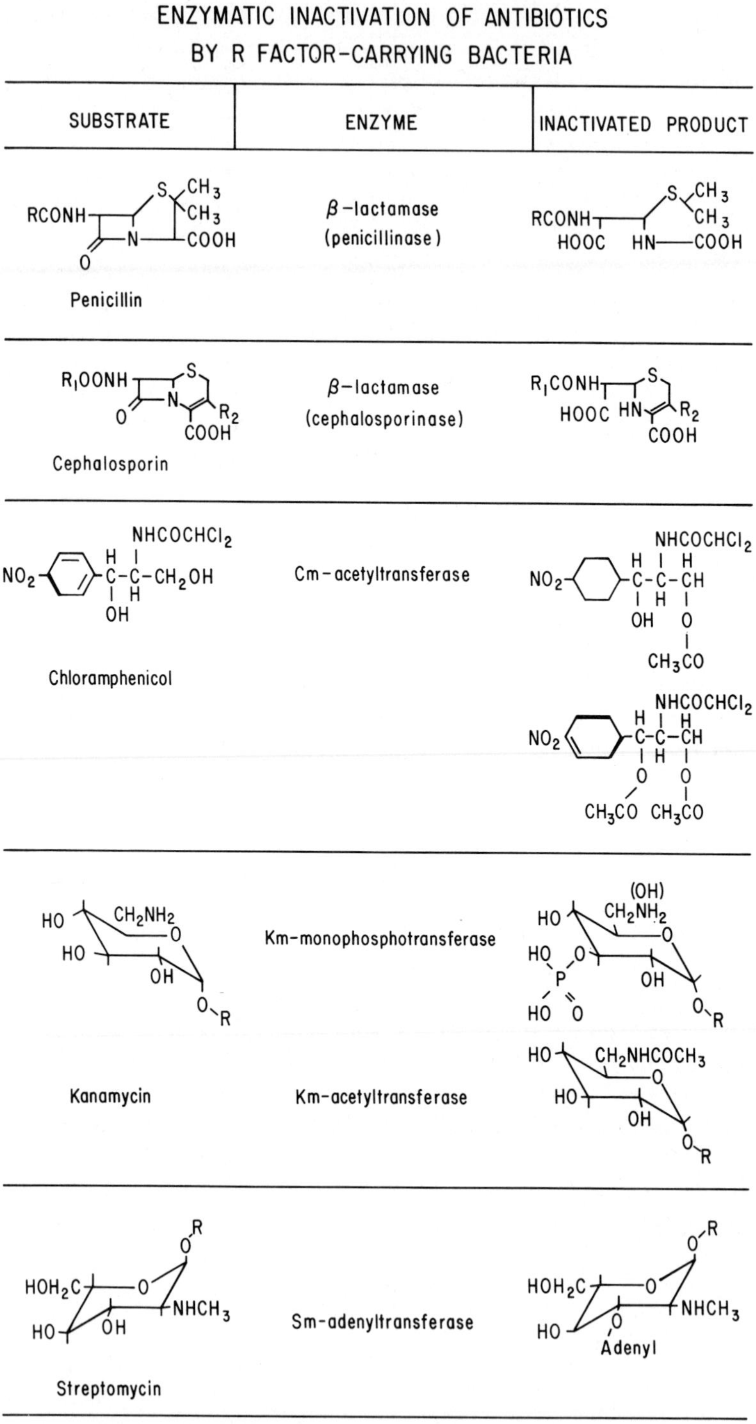

ENZYMATIC INACTIVATION OF ANTIBIOTICS
BY R FACTOR–CARRYING BACTERIA

SUBSTRATE	ENZYME	INACTIVATED PRODUCT
Penicillin	β–lactamase (penicillinase)	
Cephalosporin	β–lactamase (cephalosporinase)	
Chloramphenicol	Cm – acetyltransferase	
Kanamycin	Km–monophosphotransferase	
	Km–acetyltransferase	
Streptomycin	Sm–adenyltransferase	

Figure 4–2. Mechanisms responsible for resistance in bacteria carrying R factors. Cm = chloramphenicol; Km = kanamycin; Sm = streptomycin. (From Watanabe T: The origin of R factors. Ann NY Acad Sci *182*:131, 1971.)

ganisms. Streptomycin is by far the most important antibiotic responsible for selecting resistant mutants during treatment. Resistance develops in *E. coli* mutants because of a change in the gene that specifies the P10 protein in 30S ribosomes.[23]

The P10 protein of sensitive strains allows the attachment of streptomycin to the 30S ribosome, but in resistant strains the attachment sites for streptomycin are masked so that the drug is not bound to the ribosome. Loss of binding to the ribosome produces more or less total resistance to streptomycin and occurs in a single mutational step. Hence, there can be an abrupt appearance of resistant organisms during treatment with streptomycin after the original sensitive organisms have been rapidly eliminated. In urinary tract infections, for example, massive resistance to streptomycin can develop after five days of treatment. High-level resistance can also occur after exposure to erythromycin, apparently as a result of modification of 23S ribosomal RNA by mutation so that binding of the drug is reduced.[18] High-level resistance is not confined to drugs acting on ribosomes; it also develops to antituberculosis drugs, such as isoniazid and rifampin,[13] which do not interfere directly with ribosomal function.

Mutation appears to be responsible for gonococcal resistance to penicillin, but the level of gonococcal resistance to penicillin is much lower than that seen with streptomycin. The reason for this is that penicillin resistance does not occur in one step but increases slowly by succeeding mutational steps. Similar low-level resistance to tetracycline has occurred in gonococci, occasional strains of pneumococci, and group A streptococci.

Drug resistance can also occur in fungi and protozoa. Among fungi, resistance to 5-fluorocytosine in *Cryptococcus neoformans, Candida albicans,* and other species of *Candida* has limited the usefulness of this important new drug. High-level resistance of cryptococci and *Candida* to 5-fluorocytosine can develop by single-step mutation so that a strain sensitive to 3.0 μg/ml is no longer inhibited by 1000 μg/ml after a short period of treatment.[29]

The most important example in protozoa is the resistance to chloroquine of *Plasmodium falciparum,* the cause of malignant, subtertian malaria.[24] The major difference between chloroquine-sensitive and resistant malarial parasites is the loss of high-affinity binding of chloroquine by red blood cells infected with chloroquine-resistant parasites. Chloroquine resistance is thus attributed to a decrease in the number, affinity, or accessibility of chloroquine receptors at the site of action within the malaria parasite. The nature and subcellular location of substances that bind chloroquine are still under study.

The mechanism of acquired resistance of cryptococci or *Candida* to 5-fluorocytosine can be inferred from studies of the nonpathogenic yeast, *Saccharomyces cerevisiae.*[17] By such an analogy it has been suggested that resistance could occur through one of three processes: failure of the deamination of cytosine to 5-fluorouracil, the product responsible for blocking nucleic acid synthesis; loss of the permeases required for permeation of the drug into the yeast cell; or the absence of uracil binding sites. The first of

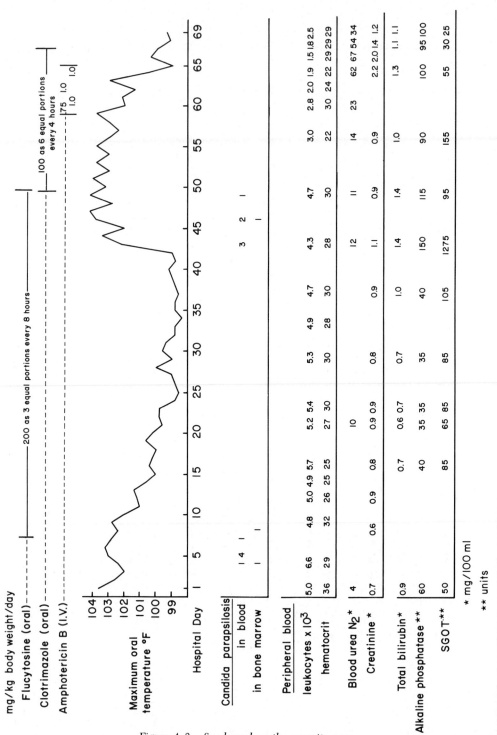

Figure 4–3. *See legend on the opposite page.*

these mechanisms, i.e., loss of cytosine deaminase activity, was responsible for acquired resistance to 5-fluorocytosine in a strain of *Candida parapsilosis* causing fatal endocarditis[15] (Fig. 4–3).

CLINICAL IMPLICATIONS OF DRUG RESISTANCE

Among antibiotic-resistant organisms, gram-negative bacteria carrying R factors present the most serious problem because their resistance to multiple drugs can be spread in epidemic proportion throughout hospitals and entire communities. In Japan the situation became so bad that in 1966–1967, 79 per cent of *Shigella* strains were resistant to one or more drugs, and at least half of these carried R factors.[20] Similar outbreaks have occurred in other parts of the world with other enteric pathogens.[3, 16, 19] In Mexico, for example, multiresistant *Salmonella typhi* recently produced the worst epidemic of typhoid fever in modern history.[12] *Shigella* and *Salmonella* resistance is primarily an epidemiologic problem outside the hospital. In hospitals as many as 60 to 70 per cent of all enteric bacteria (other than *Salmonella* and *Shigella*) carry R factors for multiple antibiotics. The high prevalence of infectious drug resistance can be traced directly to the increased use of antibiotics both in the hospital and elsewhere. The importance of selective pressure by antibiotics in promoting infectious drug resistance in hospitals can be shown by the parallel rise in resistance with drug use and by the disappearance of gram-negative bacilli transferring drug resistance when antibiotic therapy is sharply restricted.[19] Outside the hospital, when antibiotics are used in animal feed or are sold to patients without restriction, selective antibiotic pressure encourages the spread of R factors. Feed containing a penicillin or tetracycline for growth stimulation of livestock has led to the widespread distribution of enteric bacteria containing R factors. In Great Britain the extensive use of antibiotics for preventing *Salmonella* infections in cattle was followed by a human epidemic of antibiotic-resistant *Salmonella typhimurium* infection.[1] In Mexico the current epidemic of chloramphenicol-resistant typhoid fever can be related to the unrestricted sale of chloramphenicol in pharmacies to patients without prescriptions.

Although antibiotics have generated the problem, they did not create the R factor. Davis[9] has shown that R factors existed in communities that had never been exposed to commercial antibiotics (Fig. 4–4). Their evolutionary development can be explained as a survival mechanism in the presence of antibiotics produced by other organisms in the bowel or soil.

Figure 4–3. Course of illness in patient with infective endocarditis caused by *Candida parapsilosis* and treated with 5-fluorocytosine. Note relapse after the *Candida* became resistant to the drug. (From Hoeprich PD: Development of resistance to 5-fluorocytosine in *Candida parapsilosis* during therapy. J Infect Dis *130*:113, © 1974 by University of Chicago Press.)

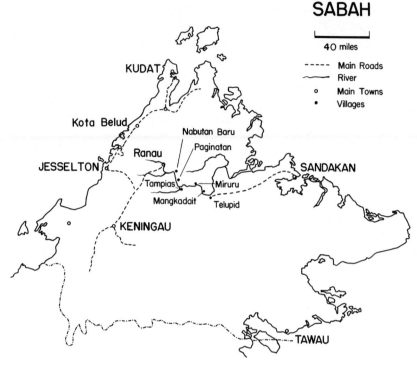

Figure 4–4. A remote locale in Borneo was used for exploring the existence of R factor before the introduction of commercial antibiotics. Davis found that R factors existed in Miruru, a community that had never been exposed to commercial antibiotics. From his discovery, it is reasonable to infer that the evolutionary development of R factor can be explained as a survival mechanism in the presence of antibiotics produced by other organisms in the bowel or soil. (From Davis CE, Anandan J: The evolution of R factor. A study of a "preantibiotic" community in Borneo. N Engl J Med 282:118, 1970.)

After the introduction of commercial antibiotics, these bacteria with R factors possessed a selective advantage and became predominant. They can transfer multiple resistance in the bowel to pathogenic enteric bacteria. Multiple resistance in one organism may involve as many as seven antibiotics. Determinants for kanamycin resistance, for example, tend to occur on R factors along with those for resistance to sulfonamides, streptomycin, tetracycline, and chloramphenicol. The use of kanamycin, therefore, could promote the simultaneous spread of resistance to itself and to four other antibiotics.[7]

Penicillinase plasmids in staphylococci have created a less serious clinical problem than the R factors in gram-negative bacteria because multiple resistance is not usually transmitted by penicillinase plasmids. Antibiotics resistant to penicillinase can therefore successfully treat infections caused by penicillinase-producing staphylococci. An exception to this is the resistance to methicillin in 10 to 17 per cent of staphylococcal infections in England, France, and Switzerland, occurring in hospitalized patients with chronic debilitating diseases.[5] This resistance may cross over to other penicillinase-resistant penicillins and is not caused by inactivation of the drug. Because they are confined to extremely debilitated patients, methicillin-resistant staphylococci have probably lost virulence even though they cause serious and even fatal infections. They are not a problem in the United States where only a few such strains have been isolated.

Chromosomal drug resistance is a major clinical problem in the treatment of tuberculosis, cryptococcosis, candidiasis, and gram-negative urinary tract infections. In cavitary pulmonary or genitourinary infections any of the antituberculosis drugs can select resistant mutants, which then produce relapses during treatment. In contrast to plasmids, which produce multiple drug resistance, chromosomal mutations affect susceptibility to only one drug. Clinical resistance, therefore, can be prevented by combination treatment with two drugs. Since the mutation rate of the tubercle bacillus to streptomycin resistance is approximately 10^{-10} and to isoniazid is 10^{-6}, the chance of developing resistance to both is only 1 in 10^{16} cell divisions. This probability is so small that the combined use of streptomycin and isoniazid in treating cavitary pulmonary tuberculosis is almost never followed by the development of resistance to either drug. This principle is also used in cryptococcosis by giving amphotericin B with 5-fluorocytosine to prevent resistance to 5-fluorocytosine; in protozoal infections to prevent trimethoprim resistance by combining trimethoprim with sulfonamides; and in E. coli urinary infections to prevent streptomycin resistance by giving streptomycin with small doses of tetracycline.

Except for these examples, chromosomal drug resistance has not been a serious clinical problem. Clinical resistance to penicillin, the most important antimicrobial, probably never occurs during the course of treating a specific infection with penicillin. Despite the high frequency of infection by penicillinase-producing staphylococci in hospitals, these organisms do not arise from penicillin-sensitive staphylococci in patients under treatment with penicillin. Their exact origin is unknown, but it is likely that penicillinase-producing staphylococci are selected out in the nasopharynx of staphylococcal carriers among hospital personnel who are exposed to low concentrations of penicillin in aerosols that develop from open vials or syringes. Penicillin resistance never occurs among pyogenic streptococci and is almost unheard of among pneumococci. The only reported exceptions are a type 23 pneumococcus isolated in 1967 from Australian patients with hypogammaglobulinemia and type 4 pneumococci recovered from 15 asymptomatic carriers in remote areas of New Guinea where penicillin was in frequent use.[14] While these strains apparently lost the extreme sensitivity to penicillin that characterizes pneumococci, they were still sensitive to 0.5 μg/ml, a level easily reached in treatment. More important, their ability to produce pneumonia or other infections has not been proved. Clinical resistance is also unheard of among infections due to Treponema pallidum, anaerobic streptococci, meningococci, leptospira, Spirillum minus, Streptobacillus moniliformis, Pasteurella multocida, and Bacillus anthracis. In other words, the vast majority of bacteria responsible for serious infections before the antibiotic era still remain fully sensitive to penicillin. Only the Staphylococcus and gonococcus are exceptions, and the genetic basis for gonococcal resistance is not yet known.

REFERENCES

1. Anderson ES: The ecology of transferable drug resistance in the enterobacteria. Annu Rev Microbiol 22:131–180, 1968.
2. Anderson ES, Datta N: Resistance to penicillins and its transfer in Enterobacteriaceae. Lancet 1:407–409, 1965.
3. Anderson ES, Smith HR: Chloramphenicol resistance in the typhoid bacillus. Br Med J 3:329–331, 1972.
4. Aserkoff B, Bennett JV: Effect of antibiotic therapy in acute salmonellosis on the fecal excretion of salmonellae. N Engl J Med 281:636–640, 1969.
5. Benner EJ, Kayser FH: Growing clinical significance of methicillin-resistant Staphylococcus aureus. Lancet 2:741–744, 1968.
6. Clowes RC: Molecular structure of bacterial plasmids. Bacteriol Rev 36:361–405, 1972.
7. Cohen S: A decade of R factors. J Infect Dis 119:104–106, 1969.
8. Datta N, Richmond MH: The purification and properties of a penicillinase whose synthesis is mediated by an R-factor in Escherichia coli. Biochem J 98:204–209, 1966.
9. Davis CE, Anandan J: The evolution of R factor. A study of a "preantibiotic" community in Borneo. N Engl J Med 282:117–122, 1970.
10. Franklin TJ: Resistance of Escherichia coli to tetracyclines. Changes in permeability to tetracyclines in Escherichia coli bearing transferable resistance factors. Biochem J 105:371–378, 1967.
11. Franklin TJ, Higginson B: The "active" accumulation of tetracycline by Escherichia coli. Biochem J 112:128, 1969.
12. Gangarosa EJ, Bennett JV, Wyatt C, et al: An epidemic-associated episome? J Infect Dis 126:215–218, 1972.
13. Guttler RB, Counts GW, Avent CK, et al: Effect of rifampin and minocycline on meningococcal carrier rates. J Infect Dis 24:199–205, 1971.
14. Hansman D, Glasgow H, Sturt J, et al: Increased resistance to penicillin of pneumococci isolated from man. N Engl J Med 284:175–177, 1971.
15. Hoeprich PD, Ingraham JL, Kleker E, et al: Development of resistance to 5-fluorocytosine in Candida parapsilosis during therapy. J Infect Dis 130:112–118, 1974.
16. Jonsson M: Antibiotic resistance and R factors in gram-negative bacteria. A study from Sweden. Scand J Infect Dis 5:Suppl:1–36, 1972.
17. Jund R, Lacroute F: Genetic and physiological aspects of resistance to 5-fluoro-pyrimidines in Saccharomyces cerevisiae. J Bacteriol 102:607–615, 1970.
18. Lai CJ, Weisblum B, Fahnestock SR, et al: Alteration of 23 S ribosomal RNA and erythromycin-induced resistance to lincomycin and spiramycin in Staphylococcus aureus. J Mol Biol 74:67–72, 1973.
19. Lowbury EJ, Babb JR, Roe E: Clearance from a hospital of gram-negative bacilli that transfer carbenicillin-resistance to Pseudomonas aeruginosa. Lancet 2:941–945, 1972.
20. Mitsuhashi S: The R factors. J Infect Dis 119:89–100, 1969.
21. Novick RP: Extrachromosomal inheritance in bacteria. Bacteriol Rev 33:210–235, 1969.
22. Okamoto S, Suzuki Y: Chloramphenicol-, dihydrostreptomycin-, and kanamycin-inactivating enzymes from multiple drug-resistant Escherichia coli carrying episome "R." Nature 208:1301–1303, 1965.
23. Ozaki M, Mizushima S, Nomura M: Identification and functional characterization of the protein controlled by the streptomycin-resistant locus in E. coli. Nature 222:333–339, 1969.
24. Peters, Wallace: Chemotherapy and Drug Resistance in Malaria. New York, Academic Press, 1970.
25. Shaw W: Enzymatic chloramphenicol acetylation and R factor induced antibiotic resistance in Enterobacteriaceae. Antimicrob Agents Chemother 221–226, 1966.
26. Shaw W: The problems of drug-resistant pathogenic bacteria. Comparative enzymology of chloramphenicol resistance. Ann NY Acad Sci 182:234–242, 1971.
27. Umezawa H, Okanishi M, Kondo S, et al: Phosphorylative inactivation of amino-glycosidic antibiotics by Escherichia coli carrying R factor. Science 157:1559–1561, 1967.
28. Watanabe T: The origin of R factors. Ann NY Acad Sci 182:126–140, 1971.
29. Weese WC: 5-Fluorocytosine therapy. Ann Intern Med 77:1003–1004, 1972.
30. Yamada T, Tipper D, Davies J: Enzymatic inactivation of streptomycin by R factor-resistant Escherichia coli. Nature 219:288–291, 1968.

CHAPTER 5

PHARMACOLOGIC PRINCIPLES

Drug efficacy is a function of concentration and antimicrobial activity in body fluids. Concentration is governed by absorption and excretion, whereas antimicrobial activity depends on protein binding and metabolic inactivation. Bioassays of body fluids for antimicrobials represent the net activity of the drug after absorption, excretion, and inactivation have occurred, and thereby give the information needed to manage an infection. For practical reasons, therefore, this chapter will deal with effective drug levels in body fluids after various routes of administration.

ABSORPTION

Table 5–1 lists the drugs that give enough absorption into the blood after oral administration to treat systemic infections. Chloramphenicol is one of the best absorbed and perhaps the only drug which obtains blood levels as good after oral as after intravenous administration.[21] Oral cephalexin, cloxacillin, and dicloxacillin also provide exceptionally high levels. As will be noted later, the high levels of cloxacillin and dicloxacillin are partly explained by low renal clearance. Cephalexin, however, is excreted rapidly by the kidneys so that its high levels are explained by excellent absorption.[15, 49] Three groups of antibiotics are notably absent from the list because of poor absorption. These are the aminoglycosides (streptomycin, kanamycin, neomycin, and gentamicin), the polymyxins (polymyxin B, colistin), and the polyenes (amphotericin B, nystatin).[33, 39, 88] Small amounts of neomycin, kanamycin, and amphotericin B may appear in the blood from the gastrointestinal tract but are not enough to rely on for therapeutic levels. All these poorly absorbed antibiotics appear to withstand the low pH of the stomach and the alkaline anaerobic environment of the bowel and can be given orally to suppress susceptible organisms. Acid lability in the stomach seems to account for the ineffectiveness of only two important antibiotics, methicillin and carbenicillin. This difficulty was solved for carbenicillin by the development of the 5-indanyl ester of car-

TABLE 5–1. *Average Serum Concentrations After Single Oral Doses in Fasting Subjects*

	Dose (mg)	Average Peak Serum Level (μg/ml)	Average Serum Half-Life (Hours)	Average Percentage Excreted in Urine in 6 Hours
Benzylpenicillin (penicillin G)	500	0.5	4.0	10.0
Phenoxymethyl penicillin (penicillin V)	500	2.9	2.0	35.0
Ampicillin	500	3.0	5.0	30.0
Amoxicillin	500	7.5	1.0	60.0
Oxacillin	500	2.6	1.5	20.0
Dicloxacillin	500	11.5	3.0	40.0
Cloxacillin	500	8.0	2.0	20.0
Indanyl carbenicillin	500	12.0	3.5	22.0
Cephalexin	500	17.0	2.0	95.0
Erythromycin base	500	1.0	3.0	0.5
Erythromycin base	250	0.35	5.5	0.5
Erythromycin stearate	500	1.1	5.0	0.5
Erythromycin stearate	250	0.4	6.0	0.5
Erythromycin estolate	500	2.5	3.5	0.9
Lincomycin	500	3.5	5.0	5.0
Clindamycin	450	4.5	3.5	5.0
Tetracycline	500	3.0	8.5	17.0
Tetracycline	250	2.2	8.0	25.0
Oxytetracycline	500	2.2	5.6	—
Chlortetracycline	500	1.4	8.0	—
Minocycline	300	4.0	15.0	2.0
Doxycycline	100	1.6	18.0	10.0
Doxycycline	200	2.8	20.0	10.0
Chloramphenicol	500	11.0	3.5	<5.0 (as active drug)
Rifampin	600	7.0	3.3	<5.0 (as active drug)
Sulfadiazine	—	—	—	7.0 (as active drug)
Sulfamethoxazole	800	53.8	12.0	10.0
Trimethoprim	160	1.58	12.0	16.0
Chloroquine	500	0.2	72.0	—
Isoniazid	600	8.5	2.6	30.0 (as active drug in 24 hr)
5-Fluorocytosine	2000	25.0	6.0	70.0 (24 hr)
Griseofulvin	500	1.25	—	<0.5
Neomycin	2000	0.95	8.0	0.85 (48 hr)
Ethambutol	1750	3.5	—	50.00 (24 hr)

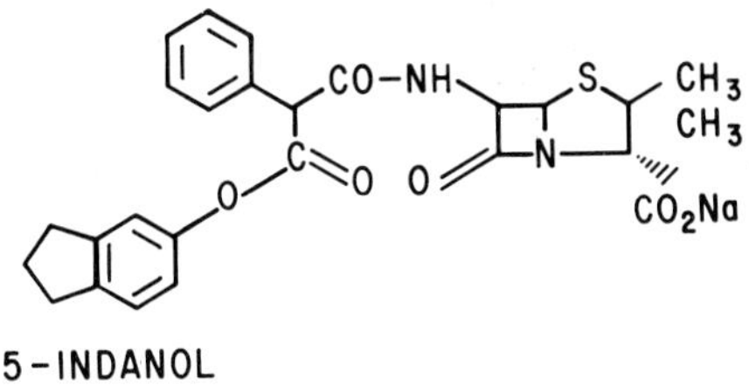

Figure 5–1. Structure of carbenicillin, the acid resistant 5-indanyl ester of carbenicillin. The α-carboxylic acid moiety of carbenicillin is bound through ester linkage to 5-indanol, and hydrolyzed after ingestion to produce active carbenicillin.

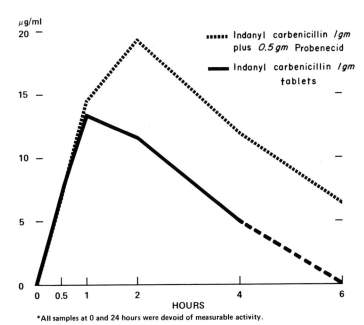

5 - INDANOL

benicillin, which is acid-resistant and well absorbed after oral administration.[13] The α-carboxylic acid moiety of carbenicillin is bound through ester linkage to 5-indanol and hydrolyzed *in vivo* to produce active carbenicillin (Figs. 5–1 and 5–2). Penicillin G (benzylpenicillin) is only slightly affected by normal gastric acidity (pH 2 to 3.5), but may be partially or totally inactivated at a pH below 2.0. For this reason potassium penicillin G is buffered with calcium carbonate or sodium phosphate for oral administration. Approximately 30 per cent of oral penicillin G is absorbed, mainly in the duodenum. Buffering is not necessary for phenoxymethyl penicillin and other

THE EFFECT OF PROBENECID, 0.5gm, ON HUMAN SERUM*
CARBENICILLIN CONCENTRATIONS (μg/ml) FOLLOWING ADMINISTRATION
OF TABLETS OF INDANYL CARBENICILLIN, /gm.

*All samples at 0 and 24 hours were devoid of measurable activity.

Figure 5–2. Carbenicillin levels after ingestion of 1.0 gm tablets of indanyl carbenicillin. These curves illustrate good absorption of active carbenicillin after hydrolysis of its 5-indanyl ester and the increased serum concentration of the antibiotic in subjects given 0.5 gm probenecid. (From Knirsch AK, Hobbs DC, Korst JJ: Pharmacokinetics, toleration, and safety of indanyl carbenicillin in man. J Infect Dis *127*:S107, © 1973 by the University of Chicago Press.)

phenoxypenicillins. Phenoxymethyl penicillin (penicillin V) has greater stability and lower solubility in acid media and is readily soluble at the alkaline pH of intestinal secretions so that it gives higher blood levels after ingestion than penicillin G.[67, 87]

Erythromycin base and erythromycin stearate are also subject to acid degradation and require protective coating or buffering to reduce destruction in the stomach. The lauryl sulfate ester of propionyl erythromycin (erythromycin estolate) withstands gastric acidity and gives better absorption than the base or stearate, but occasionally causes jaundice.[37]

Food also affects the absorption of certain oral antibiotics, but its effect is unpredictable. The absorption of cephalexin, clindamycin, and amoxicillin is not reduced by food, but most other antibiotics should be given an hour before meals to assure peak serum levels.[73, 96, 101] Such agents as aluminum hydroxide gel, magnesium sulfate, dicalcium phosphate, and iron salts should be withheld for at least one hour after the administration of tetracyclines because divalent and trivalent cations interfere with their absorption.[25] Claims that citrates, metaphosphates, glucosamines, and tetracycline phosphate complex enhance the absorption of tetracyclines have not been confirmed in well-controlled studies.[55]

The absorption of tetracyclines and lincomycin is also affected by minimal modifications of their chemical structure.[25] Conversion of lincomycin to 7-chloro-7-deoxylincomycin, or clindamycin, improves absorption after oral administration, especially in the presence of food. Among the tetracyclines, absorption increases from 25 per cent of ingested chlortetracycline to 58 per cent of oxytetracycline, 80 per cent of tetracycline, and 93 per cent of doxycycline. Doxycycline differs from oxytetracycline only by the absence of an OH group, but its absorption is almost twice as great, possibly because it is more lipophilic (Fig. 5–3). The tetracyclines are absorbed rapidly after ingestion from the duodenum to give maximum blood concentrations in one-half hour. Absorption from the stomach or ileum is much slower, however, and almost none occurs from the colon.[25, 55, 76]

In contrast to their behavior when taken orally, the aminoglycosides and polymyxins are very well absorbed after intramuscular injection. The penicillins and cephalosporin drugs are also well absorbed intramuscularly (Table 5–2). One of these, cefazolin, gives remarkably high blood levels. These levels last for eight hours and are attributed to high protein binding (86 per cent) and low renal clearance[49] (Fig. 5–4). Blood levels can be prolonged for days or weeks through the use of repository preparations that slow absorption and release penicillin slowly into the muscle depot. Benzathine penicillin G gives the most prolonged blood levels, capable of inhibiting group A streptococci and other sensitive bacteria for as long as three to four weeks. Procaine penicillin G in aqueous suspension gives effective blood levels for 48 hours after intramuscular injection of 300,000 units, and for 96 hours when suspended in oil with aluminum monostearate.

The main problems in the intramuscular route are seen with chloramphenicol, erythromycin, and tetracycline. Levels of active chloramphenicol

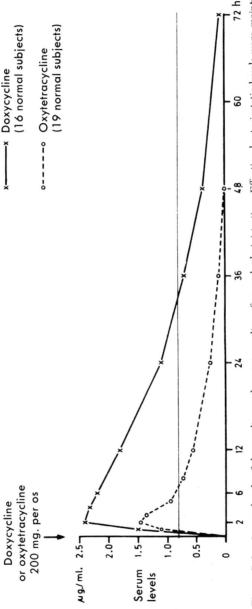

Figure 5–3. Serum levels of doxycycline and oxytetracycline after oral administration. Effective bacteriostatic levels were maintained (greater than 0.8 μg/ml) for 34 hours in the case of doxycycline and six hours in the case of oxytetracycline. (From Fabre J: Doxycycline. A Compendium of Clinical Evaluations. Pfizer Laboratories, Pfizer, Inc., 1973, p. 14.)

TABLE 5–2. *Average Serum Concentrations After Single Intramuscular Dose*

	DOSE (gm)	AVERAGE PEAK SERUM LEVEL (μg/ml)	AVERAGE SERUM HALF-LIFE (HOURS)	AVERAGE PERCENTAGE EXCRETED IN URINE IN 6 HOURS
Benzylpenicillin	0.6	12.0	0.5	70.0
Procaine penicillin G	0.2	1.0	18.0	70.0
Benzathine penicillin G	0.75	0.01	—	—
Ampicillin trihydrate	0.5	4.3	4.0	—
Sodium methicillin	1.0	16.0	1.5	66.0
Sodium oxacillin	0.5	10.9	—	—
Sodium nafcillin	0.5	—	—	10.0
Carbenicillin disodium	1.0	19.0	3.5	65.0
Sodium cephalothin	0.5	10.0	2.0	—
Sodium cefazolin	0.5	42.2	1.8	60.0
Cephaloridine	0.5	18.0	1.1	85.0 (24 hr)
Erythromycin ethylsuccinate	0.1	0.6	2.5	—
Cleocin phosphate	0.6	5.1	8.0	15.0 (24 hr)
Lincomycin hydrochloride	0.6	9.5	8.0	30.0 (24 hr)
Streptomycin	0.5	18.0	5.0	60.0 (12 hr)
Kanamycin sulfate	0.5	21.0	4.0	60.0
Gentamicin	0.06	4.7	4.0	60.0 (24 hr)
Chloramphenicol sodium succinate	1.0	5.0	6.0	1.0 (as active drug)
Polymyxin B sulfate	0.05	3.0	7.0	—
Sodium colistimethate	0.15	3.0	3.0	—
Spectinomycin	2.0	100.0	5.0	—
Pentamidine isethionate	0.280	0.5	> 24.0	15.0 (24 hr)

— = Inadequate data.
See references 8, 10, 16, 21, 28, 32, 37, 44, 46, 48–50, 71, 83, 104.

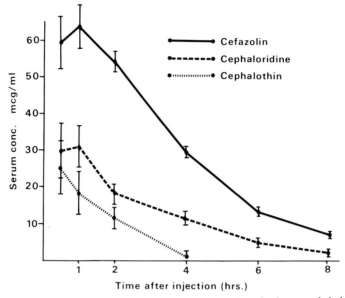

Figure 5-4. Comparison of serum concentrations of cefazolin, cephalothin, and cephaloridine after intramuscular injection of a single 1 gm dose. (From Gold JA: Experience with cefazolin: an overall summary of pharmacologic and clinical trials in man. J Infect Dis 128:S417, © 1973 by the University of Chicago Press.)

after intramuscular injection are 50 per cent of those obtained after identical oral doses because chloramphenicol succinate is not hydrolyzed to the active drug.[21] Tetracycline and erythromycin are so painful when administered intramuscularly that dosage and resulting levels are small. Pentamidine isethionate may cause pain or sterile abscesses at injection sites in a few patients but the intramuscular route is preferred because of increased systemic toxicity after intravenous injection.

EXCRETION AND INACTIVATION

Antimicrobials may be removed from the blood by the kidney, inactivated by the liver, secreted into the bile, or inactivated by other, unknown means.

Renal Excretion

The penicillins, cephalosporins, aminoglycosides, polymyxins, sulfonamides, trimethoprim, chloroquine, 5-fluorocytosine, and nitrofurantoin are eliminated primarily by the kidney as active drugs. Most tetracyclines are also excreted by the kidney. There are, however, two exceptions: chlortetracycline and minocycline are excreted mainly in the bile and feces,

TABLE 5-3. *Average Serum Concentrations After Single Intravenous Dose*

	Dose (gm)	Average Peak Serum Level (μg/ml)	Average Serum Half-Life (Hours)	Percentage of Active Drug Excreted in Urine in 6 Hours
Benzylpenicillin	0.5	5.5	0.15	90.0
Ampicillin	0.5	9.0	1.5	70.0
Sodium methicillin	0.5	16.2	0.7	80.0
Sodium oxacillin	0.5	60.0	0.4	45.0
Sodium nafcillin	0.5	40.0	0.5	35.0
Carbenicillin disodium	1.0	125.0	1.0	70.0
Sodium cephalothin	1.0	70.0	0.5	52.0 (24 hr)
Sodium cefazolin	0.5	118.0	1.8	95.0 (24 hr)
Sodium cephapirin	1.0	36.7	0.6	—
Erythromycin lactobionate	0.2	3.5	1.0	8.0
Clindamycin	0.6	8.5	3.0	20.0
Streptomycin	0.6	32.8	3.0	60.0 (12 hr)
Gentamicin sulfate	0.08	11.0	2.0	—
Sodium colistimethate	0.15	20.0	2.5	75.0
Doxycycline hyclate	0.2	4.0	18.0	71.4 (48 hr)
Tetracycline hydrochloride	0.5	8.5	8.5	45.0 (24 hr)
Oxytetracycline hydrochloride	0.5	7.0	9.2	60.0 (24 hr)
Chlortetracycline hydrochloride	0.5	9.0	5.6	15.0 (24 hr)
Amphotericin B	0.7	5.0	24.0	—
Chloramphenicol sodium succinate	1.0	11.0	3.5	5.0
Rifampin	0.6	7.0	3.3	5.0 (as active drug)
Vancomycin	0.5	33.0	6.0	80.0 (24 hr)
Sulfadiazine	—	—	—	7.0 (as active drug)
Sulfamethoxazole	0.8	53.8	10.0	10.0
Trimethoprim	0.16	1.58	10.0	16.0
Chloroquine	0.5	0.2	72.0	—
Isoniazid	0.6	8.5	6.0	30.0 (as active drug in 24 hr)
5-Fluorocytosine	2.0	25.0	6.0	70.0 (24 hr)
Griseofulvin	0.5	1.25	—	0.5

— = Inadequate data.
See references 21, 28, 30, 31, 44, 48, 50, 62, 73, 85, 93, 97, 98.

and their urinary concentrations are low.[25] Active chloramphenicol and rifampin[63] are removed mainly by the liver. Only a portion of doxycycline, erythromycin, lincomycin, and, probably, clindamycin is excreted and inactivated by the liver and kidney, and the remainder is inactivated elsewhere by unknown mechanisms. [26, 35, 45] Amphotericin B is inactivated by unknown mechanisms. Drugs excreted primarily by the kidney may be completely removed by the liver in renal insufficiency. Benzylpenicillin, for example, is inactivated at the rate of 10 per cent per hour by the liver when renal excretion fails and may not reach excessive concentrations in anuric patients.[59]

The kidney eliminates these drugs by either glomerular filtration or tubular secretion. Tubular secretion is important for the penicillins and cephalosporins, but not for other antibiotics. Only 10 per cent of benzylpenicillin is cleared by glomerular filtration and 90 per cent by tubular excretion.[22] The tubular excretion is so rapid that benzylpenicillin leaves the body more quickly than almost any other drug. When tubular excretion is less pronounced, as in the case of ampicillin, for example, renal clearance is reduced and blood levels increase. After a continuous intravenous infusion of either benzylpenicillin or ampicillin in equal amounts (0.5 gm/hour), the blood level of ampicillin is nearly twice as high and the half-life in blood twice as long.[48, 98] Carbenicillin is cleared still less slowly than ampicillin and gives correspondingly higher blood levels for longer periods of time with a given dose. Renal excretion also accounts for differences in blood levels obtained with penicillinase-resistant penicillins. Oxacillin is excreted by the kidney very rapidly and produces the lowest blood levels, while dicloxacillin, for which the renal clearance is half that of oxacillin, produces levels four times as high with the same dose (Table 5–1).

Renal clearance also accounts for differences in blood levels of the cephalosporins after intramuscular injection. Cephaloridine produces nearly twice the peak level of cephalothin because its renal clearance is twice as slow.[97] Cefazolin, in turn, has the lowest renal clearance of any cephalosporin and gives the highest peak level, equal to twice that of cephaloridine and three to four times that of cephalothin (Fig. 5–4). Cephalexin is not used parenterally but, as noted earlier, produces good peak levels by the oral route despite rapid renal elimination because the drug is so well absorbed.

Nearly all penicillins and cephalosporins are eliminated by the kidney through variable combinations of glomerular filtration and secretion by the proximal tubules. Secretion of these two groups of β-lactam drugs by the tubules is carried out by a mechanism for transporting a heterogeneous group of compounds. Many of these are carboxylic or sulfonic acids, including phenol red, hippurate, chlorothiazide, acetylated sulfonamides, and urologic contrast agents such as Diodrast. Substances secreted by this mechanism are often foreign to the body and are also eliminated by glomerular filtration.[77] In other words, the mechanism was probably evolved to secrete a toxic substance but transports nontoxic substances like penicillin because of structural similarities.

Secretion of the β-lactam antibiotics probably involves two steps. The first is from the interstitium into the proximal tubular cell, and the second from the cell into the tubular lumen. Both steps are mediated by carriers that are subject to competition for binding to the carrier. Various drugs, such as para-aminohippurate and Diodrast, have a higher affinity for the carrier system than penicillin and can block its tubular secretion, but only probenecid is used clinically for this purpose. This drug was developed during World War II when penicillin was in short supply and came from a deliberate search for an organic acid that would depress tubular secretion in order to produce high, sustained penicillin blood levels. The advantages of probenecid over other blocking drugs are its high affinity for the carrier system and its prolonged action, which results from tubular reabsorption by back diffusion and recirculation. Probenecid can block renal elimination of nearly all penicillin and cephalosporin derivatives, as well as the sulfonamides. In adequate concentration, probenecid can block completely the tubular secretion of penicillin so that renal excretion depends entirely on glomerular filtration.

Renal elimination of organic acids and bases also depends on the pH of the tubular urine. Their nonionized form is more lipid-soluble and more freely diffusible across tubular cells because of the lipid components of cell membranes. Blocking reabsorption by change in pH is more readily demonstrated with organic bases than with acids because it is easier to reduce than increase the pH of the tubular urine. For this reason, urine pH is not important in regulating excretion of the penicillins, but it has a marked influence on such organic bases as quinine, quinacrine, and chloroquine, which are eliminated more rapidly in an acid urine.

Hepatic Excretion

The liver can secrete organic acids like the penicillins, but since it cannot compete with their rapid elimination by renal tubules, biliary secretion is a minor excretory route for these antibiotics (Table 5–4). A more important hepatic function is the conversion of chloramphenicol by glucuronyltransferase to the inactive monoglucuronide, which is then se-

TABLE 5–4. *Comparative Urinary and Biliary Excretion of Antibiotics: Percentage of Administered Dose Recovered in 12 Hours*

DRUG	ROUTE	URINE	BILE
Benzylpenicillin	Intramuscular	70.0	0.08
Ampicillin	Oral	30.0	0.03
Cephaloridine	Intramuscular	85.0	0.06
Tetracycline	Oral	40.0	0.14
Erythromycin	Oral	0.5	0.04
Rifampin	Intramuscular	3.0	34.0

Source: Modified from Acocella G, Mattiussi R, Nicolis FB, et al: Biliary excretion of antibiotics in man. Gut 9:543, 1968.

creted by the renal tubules as an inactive metabolite. Only 5 to 15 per cent of chloramphenicol escapes inactivation by the liver, and this small active portion is excreted unchanged in the urine by glomerular filtration.

Other antimicrobials are probably inactivated by the liver, but the evidence is not as good as that for chloramphenicol. Rifampin, for example, is subject to desacetylation, and the desacetyl derivative accounts for all the antibiotic activity in the bile a few hours after administration. Although the site and mechanism of this transformation are unknown, hepatic enzyme changes have been demonstrated that indicate the process occurs in the liver.[14] Desacetylation causes some loss of activity against gram-positive bacteria, but not against gram-negative organisms or tubercle bacilli. Desacetylated rifampin is less readily absorbed but still re-enters the blood to produce an enterohepatic cycle that maintains prolonged blood levels. In other words, present evidence indicates that the liver transforms and excretes rifampin but does so in an active form that is reabsorbed. Hence, the ultimate elimination of the drug depends on renal excretion of 40 per cent or more and on other unknown mechanisms of inactivation.

Further evidence that desacetylation is a weak inactivating mechanism is seen with cephalothin, which has an acetyl ester at the 3-position on the cephalosporin nucleus. Cephalothin is converted by esterases, mainly in the liver, to desacetylcephalothin, while cephalexin, cephaloridine, and cefazolin do not have the acetyl ester and do not undergo this partial degradation. Removal of the acetyl group does not abolish activity against bacteria, but reduces it two- to fourfold against gram-positive organisms and

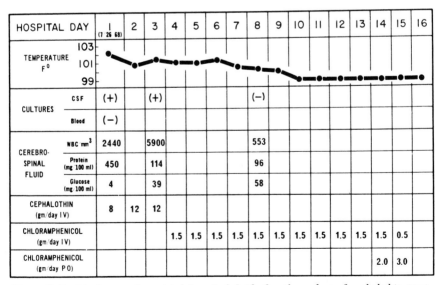

Figure 5–5. Meningococci persisted in spinal fluid after three days of cephalothin treatment. Cephalothin was then replaced by chloramphenicol, and marked clinical improvement was evident two days later. (From Southern PM Jr, Sanford JT: Meningococcal meningitis—suboptimal response to cephalothin therapy. N Engl J Med 280:1164, May 22, 1969.)

eight- to sixteenfold against gram-negative organisms.[47] Inhibition of the meningococcus requires 15 times more of the modified antibiotic. This fact may explain the failure of cephalothin in meningococcal meningitis (Fig. 5–5).

Isoniazid also appears to be transformed by the liver, but through a process of acetylation.[42] Acetyl-isoniazid is inactive and is excreted in the urine with free isoniazid. Patients fall into two distinct groups of rapid or slow inactivators, depending on the rate of acetylation. Those who inactivate isoniazid rapidly cannot be treated reliably with intermittent therapy for tuberculosis.

Most antibiotics appear in the bile and achieve the relative concentrations listed in Table 5–5.[1, 2, 26, 36, 72, 79] Rifampin is excreted in the largest amount, reaching average concentrations 100-fold greater than serum. In the absence of obstruction, nafcillin, erythromycin, and the tetracyclines can reach biliary concentrations higher than in the serum, whereas the aminoglycosides, polymyxins, most penicillins, most cephalosporins, vancomycin, and sulfonamides are excreted in the bile in small amounts. It should be noted that chloramphenicol, a drug that is totally inactivated in the liver, is excreted only slightly in the bile.

The biliary excretion of antibiotics is probably of limited clinical significance. Among those that appear in the bile in high concentrations,

TABLE 5–5. *Ratio of Antibiotic Level in Bile to Serum (Simultaneous Determinations)*

Rifampin	100.0
Erythromycin	8.0–25.0
Nafcillin	40.0
Tetracycline	5.0–10.0
Doxycycline	10.0–20.0
Oxytetracycline	6.0–10.0
Chlortetracycline	0.50–5.0
Griseofulvin	3.0
Cefazolin	3.0
Lincomycin	2.50–4.0
Streptomycin	0.40–3.0
Kanamycin	0.25–2.0
Colistin	0.60–1.0
Polymyxin B	0.60–1.0
Gentamicin	0.30–0.60
Benzylpenicillin	1.0
Ampicillin	1.0–2.0
Cephalothin	0.40–0.80
Vancomycin	0.50
Methicillin	0.20–0.50
Chloramphenicol	0.20
Cephalexin	0.16
Dicloxacillin	0.05–0.08

See references 1, 2, 35, 79.

only rifampin and the tetracyclines are active against the coliform bacteria causing infection of the biliary passages, and even their excretion is reduced by the inflammatory and obstructive processes that accompany biliary infection. Their main value might be in the prophylaxis of recurrent ascending cholangitis.

Other Mechanisms of Inactivation

The disappearance from the blood of certain antimicrobials cannot be accounted for by renal or hepatic excretion or inactivation. Amphotericin B, for example, disappears from the blood within eight hours after an intravenous injection, but less than 5 per cent of the active drug appears in the urine. The drug is probably bound to tissues and released slowly for weeks. It can be detected in the urine two months after the end of treatment.[39] Tissue binding is an important property of the tetracyclines, the polymyxins, aminoglycosides, pentamidine,[100] and quinacrine. The tetracyclines persist in tissues long after their disappearance from the serum but remain available for antimicrobial activity. In contrast, the aminoglycosides and polymyxins are inactivated by binding to tissues. Kunin's experiments[58] indicate that the polymyxins are inactivated by attachment through five free amino groups to phospholipids of cell membranes.

The disappearance from the blood of erythromycin, lincomycin, clindamycin, and doxycycline cannot be accounted for by urinary excretion, biliary excretion, or tissue binding, and large amounts (30 to 60 per cent) are thus inactivated by unknown mechanisms. The liver is usually given credit for this inactivation but without good evidence.

DISTRIBUTION

After absorption or injection into the circulation, nearly all antimicrobials are bound by serum proteins, especially albumin. The binding is normally not strong enough for hapten activity (antibody formation and hypersensitivity) and is rapidly reversible so that more drug is continually released from protein as free drug is removed. The percentage of antimicrobial drugs bound at equilibrium is indicated in Table 5–6. The clinical significance of such binding is not entirely clear, but it is claimed that binding keeps the drug from passing from the blood vessels into other body fluids, including glomerular filtrate. In other words, binding would tend to maintain blood levels at the expense of those in tissues and cerebrospinal fluids.

Binding by human serum inhibits the antimicrobial activity of antibiotics in a culture medium so that protein binding might have a deleterious effect on antibiotic activity *in vivo*. These considerations on distribution and activity should not lead to the general conclusion, however, that marked protein binding would make an antibiotic ineffective because it

TABLE 5-6. *Protein Binding of Antimicrobial Drugs (%) at Equilibrium*

Dicloxacillin	96
Cloxacillin	94
Doxycycline	82–93
Nafcillin	90
Oxacillin	90
Cefazolin	86
Phenoxymethyl penicillin	80
Cephalexin	65
Tetracycline	55–64
Cephalothin	60
Benzylpenicillin	60
Rifampin	60
Chlortetracycline	54
Colistimethate	50
Sulfadiazine	50–60
Carbenicillin	50
Methicillin	40
Streptomycin	34
Oxytetracycline	27–35
Chloramphenicol	25
Gentamicin	25
Clindamycin	25
Ampicillin	20
Cephaloridine	20
Erythromycin	18
Cephalexin	10–15
Isoniazid	0
Kanamycin	0

See references 25, 53, 54, 66, 74, 85, 91.

could not reach the infected tissues or because the concentration of free drug was too low. On the contrary, protein binding might also be viewed as chemotherapeutically favorable. Since serum proteins are selectively lost by inflammation, proteins might be regarded as a direct transport mechanism for delivering antibiotics where they are needed and for conserving the drugs from indiscriminate diffusion into, and dilution by, healthy tissue fluids and glomerular filtrate. Albumin is well suited for this function because it is smaller than other plasma proteins and therefore more accessible to the tissues during the critical early and convalescent stages of infection when capillary permeability is less marked and when antibiotics are most needed for either aborting early infections or preventing later relapse. The low specificity of albumin allows it to carry all kinds of antimicrobial drugs because it binds cations, anions, nonelectrolytes, and both aromatic and aliphatic compounds. Yet its binding affinities are small, so that free active drug is readily released into the infected fluids.

This reasoning would suggest that antibiotics bound to protein might also be retained in infected tissues after the drugs had disappeared from

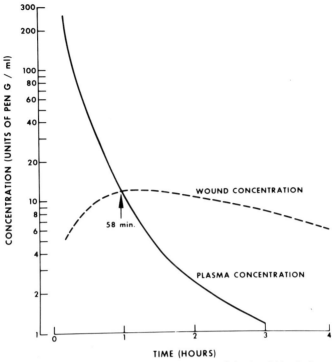

Figure 5–6. Mean concentrations of penicillin G in wound fluid and blood after intravenous injection of 100,000 units into rabbits. These curves illustrate persistence of penicillin in wounds after its disappearance from blood. (Baker G, Hunt TK: Penicillin concentrations in experimental wounds. Am J Surg *115*:532, 1968.)

the blood. In World War II, Florey found that benzylpenicillin, bound 60 per cent to protein, inhibited bacterial growth in wounds 12 hours after injection when it had disappeared from the serum. A number of studies since then have confirmed these results (Fig. 5–6). Since the protein content of inflammatory exudate approaches that of blood, 60 per cent of exudate penicillin would be held there by protein binding. Continuous infusion might not be necessary, therefore, to maintain antibiotic levels in infected tissues, and high peak levels achieved in blood with intermittent injections should produce higher concentrations in the tissues. This idea is supported by observations on penetration of antibiotics into fibrin loci *in vivo*.[4] Levels of ampicillin in fibrin clots were strikingly higher when the drug was injected intermittently than when the same total dose was given by continuous infusion, presumably because higher peak levels were reached in serum by the intermittent approach.[4] While these relationships between peak levels in serum and clot may also apply to infected tissues, the penetration of drugs into fibrin differs in other respects from the penetration into inflamed tissue. Since fibrin penetration involves gel diffusion, protein binding of antibiotics would discourage their entry. Thus, oxacillin (90 per cent protein-bound) reaches much lower levels in clots than does ampicillin (20 per cent protein-bound). In infected tissues, the inflammatory process involves the passage of protein out of the vessel into the tissues so that the protein-bound antibiotic should reach essentially the same concentration at the infected site as in serum.[12] The chief limitation of protein binding on treatment might be in bacterial endocarditis in which penetration of fibrin clots is probably needed for sterilization of the vegetation.

These ideas about the effect of protein binding on antibiotic distribution are clearly speculative. There are many discrepancies between *in vitro* observations on protein binding and the *in vivo* behavior of antibiotics, especially with respect to the predicted volume of distribution and the apparent efficacy of the drugs.[66] This is not surprising in view of the delicate techniques of dialysis or ultrafiltration needed to measure protein binding, and the many variables that affect binding. Among other things, pH is critical and the results obtained with a pH of 4.5 are completely different from those at 7.4. The lower pH of inflammatory exudate may seriously affect the release of antibiotics from protein. Other drugs and metabolites also change the protein binding of antibiotics. While protein binding undoubtedly influences the clinical action of antimicrobials along the lines discussed here, the precise effect of this phenomenon on the treatment of infection still requires considerable clarification.

The rate at which a drug leaves the circulation will also depend upon its lipid solubility, its molecular weight, and its state of aggregation. Capillaries differ in permeability. Glomerular capillaries and hepatic sinusoids are more permeable than others to molecules of all sizes, but all capillaries except those of the brain, eye, and placenta permit antimicrobials that are free in the circulation to enter the interstitial fluid readily. Most antimicrobials pass freely into pleural, ascitic, and pericardial fluids.

Central Nervous System

The permeability to antibiotics of normal capillaries in the brain is greatly reduced by tight intercellular junctions. These block intercellular passage, and antibiotics must pass through the cells rather than between them.[78] In addition, the dense capillary basement membrane is enclosed in a sheath of astrocytes. As a result, the permeability of brain capillaries resembles that of cell membranes, so that only lipid-soluble compounds enter the brain easily and rapidly. Chloramphenicol, a lipid-soluble antibiotic with low protein binding, is unique in its ability to concentrate in the brain where it produces levels nine times those in the blood (Table 5–7). On the other hand, the concentration of water-soluble antibiotics in the brain is only a small fraction of that in the blood.

A similar pattern of antibiotic distribution is seen in the cerebrospinal fluid (CSF), where the level of chloramphenicol in normal subjects is 33 to

TABLE 5–7. *Penetration of Antibiotics into Brain*

ANTIBIOTIC	AVERAGE BLOOD LEVELS (μg/ml)	AVERAGE BRAIN LEVELS (μg/gm)	BLOOD/BRAIN RATIO
Chloramphenicol	4.0	36.0	1/9
Cephalothin	11.7	1.6	7/1
Ampicillin	21.3	0.4	56/1
Penicillin	7.5	0.32	23/1
Cephaloridine	18.04	0.90	20/1

After Kramer PW, Griffith RS, Campbell RL: Antibiotic penetration of the brain. A comparative study. J Neurosurg *31*:300, 1969 Table 2.

50 per cent that of blood, while other antibiotics reach 4 per cent or less. The difference between brain and CSF levels can be partly explained by differences in the permeability of the choroid plexus and other sites of CSF formation, and by the presence of an active transport system that removes the penicillins and other drugs from the CSF.[27] The CSF is formed at the choroid plexus by a process of active secretion and flows out through the venous blood sinuses of the arachnoidal villi. Drugs may enter the CSF through the choroid plexus or from the interstitial fluid of nervous tissue and may leave by way of the venous sinuses, the capillaries of the brain and spinal cord, the choroid plexus, or the nerve cells. The concentration of a drug in the CSF represents the net result of all these factors. Entry into the CSF via choroid plexus is blocked by continuous tight junctions between the choroidal cells, so that a substance moving from the blood into the CSF goes freely *between* the capillary endothelial cells of the plexus, but must pass *through* the choroidal epithelial cells. Consequently, entry into the CSF is governed by the same factors that limit passage through the brain capillaries: molecular size, protein binding, lipid solubility, and ionization. Again, these factors favor the passage of chloramphenicol but not of the water-soluble antibiotics. The short-acting sulfonamides, such as sulfadiazine (which is only 22 per cent protein-bound) and isoniazid, also pass readily into the CSF. The penicillins not only have trouble passing the normal blood-brain barrier into the CSF but tend to be removed rapidly by active transport from the CSF to the blood. Since transport out can be blocked by probenecid, the drug might enhance the effect of penicillin in meningitis.[89] Probenecid would also produce higher blood levels of penicillins by the inhibition of renal and biliary excretion, and reduce protein binding of penicillin by competing for serum protein. On the other hand, probenecid might have an adverse effect on brain infections because it competes with penicillin for entry into the brain.

The drug therapy of meningitis benefits from a generalized nonspecific increase in membrane permeability and a decreased removal of large molecules by the arachnoidal villi, so that CSF/blood antibiotic ratios are increased. Yow reported, for example, that ampicillin can produce mean CSF levels of 0.8 μg/ml in normal subjects with blood levels of 24.9 μg/ml, a CSF/blood ratio of 4.4 per cent. She found that in viral meningitis the mean

CSF level rose to 1.2 with blood levels of 17.7 (ratio, 9.1 per cent) and that in bacterial meningitis the mean CSF level reached 1.9 μg/ml with blood levels of 15 μg/ml (ratio, 12.7 per cent). This rise in CSF/blood ratio from 4.4 to 12.7 per cent in bacterial meningitis produced adequate CSF levels for the treatment of pneumococcal, meningococcal, and *H. influenzae* meningitis.[3] Similar increases in CSF/blood ratios with meningitis have been reported with methicillin, cephalothin, cephaloridine, penicillin, rifampin, lincomycin, carbenicillin, the tetracyclines, and sulfonamides so that all these drugs may be used successfully in treating certain forms of meningitis. Meningitis improves CSF penetration of the aminoglycosides, but not enough to treat gram-negative bacillary infections, and these drugs must be injected intrathecally to cure meningitis. Since adequate CSF levels of erythromycin cannot be achieved by any route, this drug has no place in the treatment of meningitis. Perhaps the highest CSF/blood ratios are obtained with 5-fluorocytosine. In cryptococcal meningitis the CSF levels of 5-fluorocytosine are 75 per cent those in serum.[9] Isoniazid and trimethoprim are also able to achieve therapeutic levels in the CSF during meningitis.

Placenta

Although the membranes separating fetal capillary blood from maternal blood should impose the same restriction to drug passage that exists in the brain and choroid plexus, water-soluble antibiotics freely enter the fetal circulation if they are not bound heavily to protein. Most studies on drug passage are conducted by comparing levels in cord blood and maternal blood at term when the thickness and number of layers interposed between fetal and maternal blood are reduced to a minimum, while the absorbing surface area is increased. These changes in the fetal-maternal barrier may account for the fact that water-soluble drugs with low protein binding (20 to 40 per cent), such as ampicillin and methicillin, reach nearly the same peak

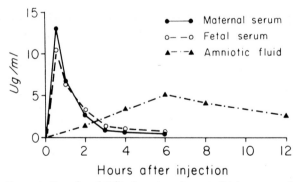

Figure 5–7. Concentration of methicillin in maternal serum, fetal serum, and amniotic fluid. This water-soluble drug with low protein binding readily passes the placental barrier at term and produces nearly the same peak level in fetal serum as in maternal serum. (From Depp R, et al: Transplacental passage of methicillin and dicloxacillin into the fetus and amniotic fluid. Am J Obstet Gynecol *107*:1056, 1970.)

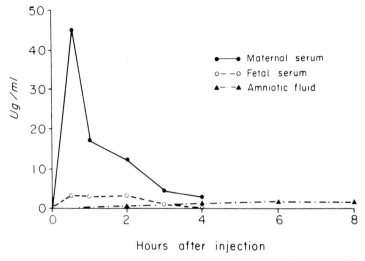

Figure 5–8. Concentration of dicloxacillin in maternal serum, fetal serum, and amniotic fluid. This drug is highly bound to protein (95 per cent) and passes the placental barrier poorly. (From Depp R, et al: Transplacental passage of methicillin and dicloxacillin into the fetus and amniotic fluid. Am J Obstet Gynecol *107*:1056, 1970.)

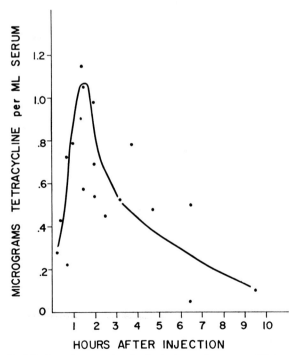

Figure 5–9. Umbilical cord serum levels illustrate good passage of tetracycline into fetal circulation. The umbilical cord serum level reaches 60 per cent of the maternal level. The peak amniotic fluid level of tetracycline is about 50 per cent of the cord serum level. (From Le Blanc AL, Perry JE: Transfer of tetracycline across the human placenta. Texas Rep Biol Med 25:543, 1967.)

level at term in fetal serum as in maternal serum within 30 to 60 minutes after intravenous injection (Fig. 5–7). However, after injection of dicloxacillin, which is 95 per cent bound to protein, the fetal/maternal peak serum ratio is only 7 per cent, and peak concentrations in amniotic fluid are less than 5 per cent[19] (Fig. 5–8). Benzylpenicillin, the tetracyclines (Fig. 5–9), lincomycin, streptomycin, the cephalosporins, sulfonamides, chloramphenicol, and isoniazid all reach effective levels in fetal blood with penetration up to 75 per cent of maternal levels or greater in 90 minutes. Therapeutic concentrations of the cephalosporins and lincomycins are also found in amniotic fluid, but only negligible amounts of streptomycin, tetracycline, and chloramphenicol are found there.[20] For this reason, and in view of their toxicity to the fetus, the last three should not be used in pregnancy. Among antiprotozoal drugs, quinine, primaquine, and metronidazole readily pass the placenta, but there is little published data concerning fetal toxicity, and they should be used cautiously.

Eye

The passage of antibiotics from the blood into the eye also encounters a barrier. Studies are limited in man, but from experimental data on rabbits and a few observations of patients undergoing cataract extraction, it appears that chloramphenicol gives the best levels in the aqueous. After parenteral administration of most other antibiotics, the level in the aqueous may be sufficient to treat infection due to sensitive bacteria only. Peak levels in the aqueous of human eyes reach 0.3 μg/ml penicillin after 600 mg IM and 0.55 μg/ml cephalothin, 2.5 to 17.0 μg/ml cephaloridine, and 1.0 μg ampicillin[80] after 1.0 gm IV. After two tablets of trimethoprim (80 mg)–sulfamethoxazole (400 mg) were given orally twice daily to patients with cataracts, both drugs reached therapeutically effective amounts in the aqueous.[77a] The concentration of trimethoprim ranged from 0.14 to 40 μg/ml, and for sulfamethoxazole it ranged from 10 to 29 μg/ml. Methicillin does not penetrate into the aqueous of normal noninflamed human eyes in therapeutic amounts, even when high blood levels are obtained, but may reach effective levels against staphylococci in severely inflamed eyes. The blood-aqueous barrier is probably altered by inflammation. No significant penetration of any antibiotic into the normal vitreous occurs in rabbits, but human vitreous penetration has not been studied.

After subconjunctival injection, ampicillin penetrates aqueous humor in bactericidal concentrations against E. coli, and both ampicillin and penicillin reach bacteriostatic concentrations against S. aureus. Chloramphenicol succinate and streptomycin did not penetrate aqueous humor in effective concentrations in one study of the subconjunctival route,[70] but a 0.5 per cent solution of chloramphenicol gave aqueous humor levels of 3.5 to 6.7 μg/ml when applied topically to patients two to five hours before cataract surgery.[5]

Synovial Fluid

Most antibiotics enter infected joints so well that intra-articular injections are unnecessary. Penicillin G, penicillin V, ampicillin, methicillin, cephalothin, cloxacillin, nafcillin, cephaloridine, tetracycline, lincomycin, and gentamicin all reach levels in infected joints approaching or exceeding those in serum[75] (Fig. 5–10). Limited observations suggest that erythromycin and the polymyxins may not be transported from the blood into infected joints in therapeutic concentrations.

Pleural, Pericardial, and Ascitic Fluids

Most antibiotics, including erythromycin and the sulfonamides, pass freely into infected serous cavities where they usually reach levels of 50 per cent or more of those found in serum.

Ear and Paranasal Sinuses

Thirty minutes after IM injection in acute otitis, penicillin in middle ear secretions is 15 per cent of the serum level. It rises to 40 per cent in an hour and equilibrates with serum at six hours. After 12 hours the penicillin

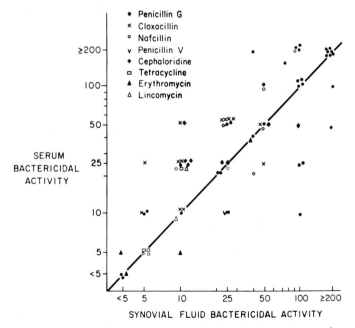

Figure 5–10. Comparison of the bactericidal levels of antibiotics in 75 paired serum and synovial fluids during systemic antibiotic therapy. Points on the diagonal line indicate pairs with equal activity. Bactericidal activity is expressed as the reciprocal of the maximum dilution showing this activity. (From Parker RH, Schmid F: Antibacterial activity of synovial fluid during therapy of septic arthritis. Arthritis Rheum *14*:99, 1971.)

concentration is higher in ear secretion than in serum.[41, 61] In chronic otitis, on the other hand, the penicillin concentration is very low and often undetectable, possibly because the bacteria in chronic infections produce penicillinase. Ampicillin, tetracycline, erythromycin, and sulfonamides also pass into the ear freely in acute otitis media in concentrations that inhibit sensitive organisms.

Penicillin reaches therapeutic levels in the mucosa of the paranasal sinuses, but not as consistently as tetracycline. In the maxillary sinus, for example, the usual mucosal/serum concentration ratio of penicillin is between 0.5 and 1, while that for tetracycline is 1 or more.[65] For erythromycin the ratio is between 0.4 and 0.8 in patients given erythromycin stearate orally.[44]

Prostate

A blood-prostate barrier, comparable to that in the brain, keeps most antimicrobials out of the gland under normal conditions and during chronic infection because of lipid insolubility, protein binding, and a high degree of ionization in plasma.[90] Certain sulfonamides and erythromycin are exceptions and seem to penetrate the normal gland, but usually lack activity against the organisms that cause chronic prostatitis. There is evidence that doxycycline and trimethoprim, perhaps because of their lipophilic character, reach the same or higher levels in the prostate as in the serum and may prove valuable in treatment of chronic prostatitis.[29, 90] Therapeutic results in acute prostatitis indicate that the inflammatory changes alter the barrier and allow most antibiotics to penetrate.

Kidney

Antibiotics excreted in urine reach concentrations many times greater than in serum, but their distribution in the kidney parenchyma has received little study. The mean urinary concentrations of penicillin G, for example, regularly exceed 100 μg/ml, with serum levels less than 0.5 μg/ml in normal subjects taking 500 mg of penicillin G orally every six hours before eating. Since most strains of E. coli, Proteus, and enterococci are killed at these concentrations, penicillin can be used to treat bacilluria even though the drug would be ineffective against these organisms in other body fluids. Similarly, in adults receiving 250 mg tetracycline or oxytetracycline, the urinary concentrations of these two drugs are well over 100 μg/ml while serum levels are only 1 to 2 μg/ml. In general, these concentrations are those predicted from the proportion of active drug excreted in the urine (see Table 5–3), and such estimates can be made for other antimicrobials from a knowledge of active drug and urine excretion rates. The importance of urine levels in treating kidney infections probably depends on two factors. First, elimination of bacteria from the urine removes the source for reinfection of the kidney. Second, intrarenal concentration of the drug might be a function of its level in the tubular urine. There is little information on either point, although claims have been made

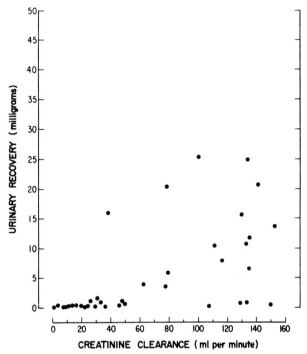

Figure 5–11. Impaired excretion of nitrofurantoin in renal failure is illustrated by recovery of no drug two hours after a single oral dose of 100 mg in patients with depressed creatinine clearance. (From Sachs J, Geer T, Noell P, Kunin CM: Effect of renal function on urinary recovery of orally administered nitrofurantoin. N Engl J Med 278:1033, 1968.)

that the cure of kidney infections depends on urinary, rather than serum, drug levels.[103] The limited data on intrarenal distribution of antimicrobial drugs suggest that ampicillin and certain other antibiotics reach concentrations in the cortex that are twice those in the medulla or papilla and eight times the serum level.[103] In pyelonephritis and other renal disease the situation appears to be reversed so that levels in kidney tissue are only one-half those in serum. This decline in drug level in the diseased kidney occurs with both carbenicillin and ampicillin, and probably results from poor diffusion into diseased tissue and impaired renal concentration. The urinary levels also decline markedly, so that the normal advantage of urinary excretion and concentration of certain antibiotics is lost, and effective drug levels in the diseased kidney must be calculated from serum concentrations instead. At least one drug, nitrofurantoin, does not appear in the urine in severe renal failure and is contraindicated in azotemic patients[84] (Fig. 5–11).

RENAL FAILURE

The delay in excretion of antibiotics in renal failure is reflected in their longer half-life in serum and reduced levels in urine. The aminoglycosides,

TABLE 5–8. *Half-Life (Hours)*

	NORMAL	EXTREME RENAL FAILURE (CREATININE CLEARANCE < 5 ml/min)	REMOVAL BY PERITONEAL DIALYSIS (%)	REMOVAL BY HEMO-DIALYSIS (%)
Vancomycin	6.0	218.0	—	0
Tetracycline HCl	8.5	57.0–108.0	slight	0
Kanamycin	4.0	48.0–96.0	40.0	70.0
		(3 × serum creatinine)		
Streptomycin	2.0–3.0	52.0–110.0	—	—
Gentamicin	2.0–3.0	67.0 (4 × creatinine)	5.0–50.0	80.0
Polymyxin B	7.0	72.0	0	0
Colistimethate	4.5	10.3	15.0	0
Minocycline	13.0	35.0	0	0
Oxytetracycline	9.3	48.0–66.0	0	0
Cefazolin	2.0	35.0	0	25.0
Cephalexin	2.0	20.0	—	75.0
Cephalothin	0.5	2*/16**	2.0	90.0
Carbenicillin	1.0	14.0	50.0	80.0
Ampicillin	0.5	13.0	0	80.0
Lincomycin	4.0	11.0	0	0
Clindamycin	2.4	10.0	10.0	—
Doxycycline	15.0–20.0	15.0–20.0	0	0
Chlortetracycline	5.6	7.0–11.0	slight	0
Benzylpenicillin	0.15	7.2–10.5	0	slight
Methicillin	0.7	4.0	0	slight
Oxacillin	0.4	2.0	0	slight
Erythromycin	1.4	5.0	0	0
Rifampin	3.3	4.0	—	—
Isoniazid	2.6	4.3	?	?
Amphotericin B	24.0	?	0	0
Chloramphenicol	1.6–3.3	3.2–4.3	0	0
5-Fluorocytosine	4.0–8.0	30.0–250.0	—	50.0
Trimethoprim	12.0	24.0	—	0
Sulfamethoxazole	12.0	>24.0	—	0

* = Cephalothin.
** = Desacetylcephalothin.
— = Inadequate data.
See references 6, 17, 23, 26, 40, 43, 47, 52, 53, 56, 64, 69, 74, 81, 99, 102.

polymyxins, and vancomycin, which are excreted almost entirely by the kidney, persist the longest in the serum in extreme renal failure (Table 5–8). One can calculate aminoglycoside serum half-lives as a multiple of creatinine by correlating the excretion rates of creatinine and these antibiotics.[18] The half-life of kanamycin is approximately three times the serum creatinine level, and for gentamicin it is equal to four times the creatinine (Fig. 5–12). Since a dose of kanamycin (7 mg/kg) given every third half-life will maintain an effective drug level, the dosage interval is nine times the serum creatinine level. The dosage interval needed to maintain an effective

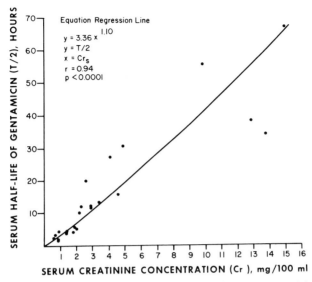

Figure 5–12. Relation of serum half-life of gentamicin (T½) to serum creatinine concentration in 24 patients. (From McHenry MC, Gavan TL, Gifford RW Jr, et al: Gentamicin dosages for renal insufficiency. Ann Intern Med 74:194, 1971.)

level of gentamicin (1.3 mg/kg) is every second half-life, so that the dosage interval would be eight times the serum creatinine.[69]

Similar guidelines based on prolonged serum half-life are available for other drugs, although formulas related to creatinine are limited to kanamycin and gentamicin. The half-life of vancomycin is prolonged to nine days in anuric patients, and a dose of 1 gm is required every seven days to maintain effective levels against staphylococci.[24] Colistimethate requires a progressive reduction in dosage with increasing levels of creatinine.[34] As the creatinine clearance approaches 20 ml/minute, the normal daily dose of 5 mg/kg is reduced to 4.0 mg/kg; below 20 ml/minute to 2.5 mg/kg; and below 5 ml/minute to 1.5 mg/kg.

The only other antimicrobials that persist in excessive amounts for days in the circulation during extreme renal failure are 5-fluorocytosine and certain members of the tetracycline group. In anuria the half-life of tetracycline hydrochloride is four to five days, oxytetracycline two to three days, and minocycline one and one-half days. The half-life of doxycycline in the serum is not affected by renal failure, because renal insufficiency is accompanied by accelerated inactivation even though urinary clearance of the drug diminishes as a direct function of glomerular filtration.[26] Chlortetracycline also shows little tendency to accumulate during renal insufficiency because of increased metabolic conversion and biliary excretion[26] (Fig. 5–13). All tetracyclines except doxycycline aggravate the elevation of blood urea nitrogen in renal insufficiency. For these reasons, most tetracyclines are not given to patients with severe renal failure, since doxycycline can be used instead.

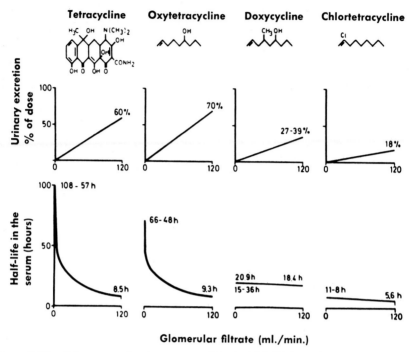

Figure 5-13. Urinary excretion (percentage of dose) and half-life in the serum of tetracyclines as a function of glomerular filtration. (From Fabre J: Doxycycline, A Compendium of Clinical Evaluations. Pfizer Laboratories, Pfizer, Inc., 1973, p. 24.)

The penicillins and cephalosporins are usually not a serious problem in renal failure because hepatic inactivation and excretion can compensate to a large extent for failure of renal excretion, and because even high levels of these drugs are not usually dangerous. One-half the usual dose can be given each half-life, after the loading dose, to anuric patients. Kunin points out that this simple method provides peak levels equal to those obtained in individuals with normal kidneys and will ensure high blood levels between doses.[53] This means that a drug like cefazolin, usually given in doses of 500 mg every eight hours to provide average peak serum levels of 42.2 μg/ml, would be given to uremic patients in a starting dose of 500 mg followed by 250 mg at 36-hour intervals.[15]

Most other antibiotics can be given without adjusting the dose in renal failure. Doxycycline, chlortetracycline, isoniazid, erythromycin, amphotericin B, and rifampin require no significant adjustment in dosage. Minor adjustments are needed for clindamycin and lincomycin.[81]

Dosage in uremia is also affected by dialysis. Hemodialysis removes large amounts of the aminoglycosides (Fig. 5-14) and of certain β-lactam drugs; namely, ampicillin, carbenicillin (Fig. 5-15), cephalothin, and cephalexin. Peritoneal dialysis lowers the serum level of carbenicillin and of the aminoglycosides about 50 per cent. The portion of drug removed by dialysis should be replaced by a dose of the same proportion. For example,

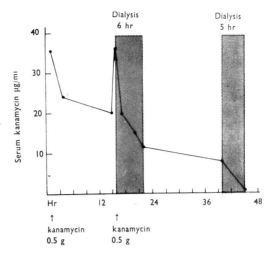

Figure 5–14. The effect of hemodialysis on the serum levels of kanamycin in a patient with oliguric renal failure. Hemodialysis caused prompt and significant falls in the serum levels of kanamycin. (From Altmann G, et al: Blood levels of ampicillin, kanamycin and gentamicin in the uremic patient. Isr J Med Sci 6:688, 1970.)

if 70 per cent of kanamycin is removed, it should be replaced upon completion of dialysis by 70 per cent of the standard dose.

Not only the antibiotics, but the antifolic drugs, trimethoprim and sulfamethoxazole, also accumulate in the serum of patients with renal failure. The usual combination tablet sold commercially contains 80 mg trimethoprim and 400 mg sulfamethoxazole, and each of the two drugs has a normal half-life of about 12 hours in the serum. When the creatinine clearance falls below 30 ml/minute, the interval between doses of two tablets should be increased from 12 to 24 hours, and below 15 ml/minute,

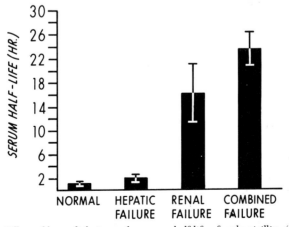

Figure 5–15. Effect of hemodialysis on the serum half-life of carbenicillin. (From Hoffman TA, Cestero R, Bullock WE: Pharmacokinetics of carbenicillin in patients with hepatic and renal failure. J Infect Dis *122*:S76, © 1970 by the University of Chicago Press.)

TABLE 5–9. *Effect of Hemodialysis on Sulfadiazine Blood Levels (mg/100 ml)*

	DOSAGE	BEFORE DIALYSIS	AFTER DIALYSIS
Case 1	1.5 gm daily + 1.0 gm after each dialysis	6.2	2.2
	2.0 gm daily + 1.5 gm after each dialysis	13.5	7.4
Case 2	1.0 gm daily	13.5	6.0
	1.5 gm daily	14.5	6.0

"Free" sulfadiazine levels in two cases of nocardiosis in renal transplant patients who improved on sulfadiazine therapy. Free (active drug) levels are usually two-thirds or more of total. Inactive drug is acetylated. Levels of 8 to 20 mg/100 ml of free drug are usually needed for cure of pulmonary nocardiosis. (Case 1 courtesy of Dr. George Pazin; case 2 courtesy of Dr. Elizabeth Ziegler.)

the drugs should not be used.[7] Even with marked loss of renal function, the urine levels of trimethoprim and sulfamethoxazole always exceed the effective therapeutic concentration for urinary bacteria.[86]

The relationship between serum levels, serum half-life, and renal insufficiency is not very clear for the other sulfonamides, and levels must be monitored if the sulfonamides are used in renal failure, as might be necessary if, for example, nocardiosis should develop in transplant cases receiving adrenal steroids (Table 5–9).

Monitoring of serum levels is a prerequisite for the use of all antimicrobials in renal failure, even when the pharmacology has been well worked out. Most of the formulations presented here are based on a small number of studies in a limited number of patients and must be regarded only as approximate guidelines for treatment. The need for careful assays of antimicrobials in renal failure, especially of toxic drugs capable of heavy accumulation, cannot be emphasized too strongly.

HEPATIC INSUFFICIENCY

Antibiotics metabolized or excreted by the liver can reach higher levels than normal in patients with severe liver disease. The serum levels and half-lives of rifampin, isoniazid, lincomycin, and unconjugated chloramphenicol are significantly higher in patients with chronic impairment of hepatic function. The occurrence of hepatic disease in renal failure may further prolong the half-lives of antibiotics like the penicillins and cephalosporins that are excreted or metabolized by the liver when their primary excretory route through the kidney no longer functions (Fig. 5–16). Toxic effects from chloramphenicol may take the form of depressed erythropoiesis and encephalopathy when hepatic function is severely de-

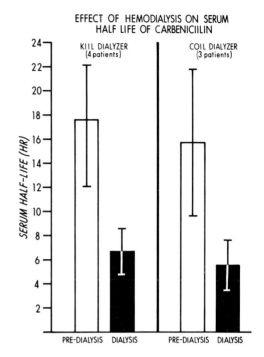

EFFECT OF HEMODIALYSIS ON SERUM
HALF LIFE OF CARBENICIILIN

Figure 5–16. Effect of hepatic dysfunction, oliguric renal failure, and combined hepatorenal failure upon the mean serum half-life of carbenicillin after a single 2 gm intravenous dose. (From Hoffman TA, Cestero R, Bullock WE: Pharmacokinetics of carbenicillin in patients with hepatic and renal failure. J Infect Dis *122*:S76, © 1970 by the University of Chicago Press.)

pressed, but the role of hepatic dysfunction in producing toxicity from other antibiotics has not been clearly demonstrated.[94]

REFERENCES

1. Acocella G, Mattiussi R, Nicolis FB, et al: Biliary excretion of antibiotics in man. Gut 9:536–545, 1968.
2. Ayliffe GA, Davies A: Ampicillin levels in human bile. Br J Pharmacol *24*:189–193, 1965.
3. Barrett FF, Eardley WA, Yow MD, et al: Ampicillin in the treatment of acute suppurative meningitis. J Pediatr 69:343–353, 1966.
4. Barza M, Brusch J, Bergeron M, et al: Penetration of antibiotics into fibrin loci in vivo. III. Intermittent vs. continuous infusion and the effect of probenecid. J Infect Dis *129*:73–78, 1974.
5. Beasley H, Boltralik JJ, Baldwin HA: Chloramphenicol in aqueous humor after topical application. Arch Ophthalmol 93:184–185, 1975.
6. Bennett WM, Singer I, Coggins CH: Guide to drug usage in adult patients with impaired renal function. A supplement. JAMA *223*:991–997, 1973.
7. Bergan T, Brodwall EK: Human pharmacokinetics of a sulfamethoxazole-trimethoprim combination. Acta Med Scand *192*:483–492, 1972.
8. Black J, Calesnick B, Williams D, et al: Pharmacology of gentamicin, a new broad-spectrum antibiotic. Antimicrob Agents Chemother 138–147, 1963.
9. Block ER, Bennett JE: Pharmacologic studies with 5-fluorocytosine. Antimicrob Agents Chemother *1*:476–482, 1972.
10. Boger WP, Gavin JJ: Kanamycin: its cerebrospinal fluid diffusion, renal clearance, and comparison with streptomycin. Antibiot Annu 677–683, 1958–59.
11. Bond JM, Lightbown JW, Barber M, et al: A comparison of four phenoxypenicillins. Br Med J 2:956–961, 1963.
12. Brown DM: Tissue distribution of penicillins. Postgrad Med J Suppl *40*:31–36, 1964.

13. Butler K, English A, Knirsch A, Korst J: Metabolism and laboratory studies with indanyl carbenicillin. *In* Infectious Disease Reviews. Edited by Holloway WJ. Wil² mington, Futura Publishing Co., 1972, pp. 157–166.

14. Cohn HD: Clinical studies with a new rifamycin derivative. J Clin Pharmacol 9:118–125, 1969.

15. Craig WA, Welling PG, Jackson TC, et al: Pharmacology of cefazolin and other cephalosporins in patients with renal insufficiency. J Infect Dis 128:Suppl:S347–353, 1973.

16. Cronk GA, Naumann DE: The absorption and excretion of kanamycin in human beings. J Lab Clin Med 53:888–895, 1959.

17. Cutler RE, Gyselynck AM, Fleet WP, et al: Correlation of serum creatinine concentration and gentamicin half-life. JAMA 219:1037–1041, 1972.

18. Cutler RE, Orme BM: Correlation of serum creatinine concentration and kanamycin half-life. Therapeutic implications. JAMA 209:539–542, 1969.

19. Depp R, Kind AC, Kirby WM, et al: Transplacental passage of methicillin and dicloxacillin into the fetus and amniotic fluid. Am J Obstet Gynecol 107:1054–1057, 1970.

20. Duignan NM, Andrews J, Williams JD: Pharmacological studies with lincomycin in late pregnancy. Br Med J 3:75–78, 1973.

21. DuPont HL, Hornick RB, Weiss CF, et al: Evaluation of chloramphenicol acid succinate therapy of induced typhoid fever and Rocky Moutain spotted fever. N Engl J Med 282:53–57, 1970.

22. Eagle H, Newman E: Renal clearance of penicillins F, G, K, and X in rabbits and man. J Clin Invest 26:903–918, 1947.

23. Eastwood JB, Curtis JR: Carbenicillin administration in patients with severe renal failure. Br Med J 1:486–487, 1968.

24. Eykyn S, Phillips I, Evans J: Vancomycin for staphylococcal shunt site infections in patients on regular haemodialysis. Br Med J 3:80–82, 1970.

25. Fabre J, Milek E, Kalfopoulos P, et al: The kinetics of tetracyclines in man. I. Digestive absorption and serum concentrations. *In* Doxycycline, A Compendium of Clinical Evaluations. New York, Pfizer Laboratories Division, Pfizer Inc., 1973, pp. 13–18.

26. Fabre J, Milek E, Kalfopoulos P, et al: The kinetics of tetracyclines in man. II. Excretion, penetration in normal inflammatory tissues, behavior in renal insufficiency and hemodialysis. *In* Doxycycline, A Compendium of Clinical Evaluations. New York, Pfizer Laboratories Division, Pfizer Inc., 1973, pp. 19–28.

27. Fishman RA: Blood-brain and CSF barriers to penicillin and related organic acids. Arch Neurol (Chicago) 15:113–124, 1966.

28. Froman J, Gross L, Curatola S: Serum and urine levels following parenteral administration of sodium colistimethate to normal individuals. J Urol 103:210–214, 1970.

29. Garnes HA: Doxycycline levels in serum and prostatic tissue in man. Urology 1:205–207, 1973.

30. Geraci JE, Heilman FR, Nichols DR, et al: Some laboratory and clinical experiences with a new antibiotic, vancomycin. Antibiot Annu 90:106, 1956–1957.

31. Gilbert DN, Sanford JP: Methicillin: critical appraisal after a decade of experience. Med Clin North Am 54:1113–1125, 1970.

32. Gingell JC, Waterworth PM: Dose of gentamicin in patients with normal renal function and renal impairment. Br Med J 2:19–22, 1968.

33. Goodwin NJ: Colistin and sodium colistimethate. Med Clin North Am 54:1267–1276, 1970.

34. Goodwin NJ, Friedman EA: The effects of renal impairment, peritoneal dialysis, and hemodialysis on serum sodium colistimethate levels. Ann Intern Med 68:984–994, 1968.

35. Griffith RS, Black HR: A comparison of blood levels after oral administration of erythromycin and erythromycin estolate. Antibiot Chemother 12:398–403, 1962.

36. Griffith RS, Black HR: Cephalexin: a new antibiotic. Clin Med 75(11):14–22, 1968.

37. Griffith RS, Black HR: Erythromycin. Med Clin North Am 54:1199–1215, 1970.

38. Hammerstrom CF, Cox F, McHenry MC, et al: Clinical, laboratory, and pharmacological studies of dicloxacillin. Antimicrob Agents Chemother 69–74, 1966.

39. Hildick-Smith G: Antifungal antibiotics. Pediatr Clin North Am 15:107–118, 1968.

40. Hoffman TA, Cestero R, Bullock WE: Pharmacokinetics of carbenicillin in patients with hepatic and renal failure. J Infect Dis 122:Suppl:S75–77, 1970.

41. Howie VM, Ploussard JH: The "in vivo sensitivity test"—bacteriology of middle ear exudate, during antimicrobial therapy in otitis media. Pediatrics 44:940–944, 1969.
42. Hughes HB: On the metabolic fate of isoniazid. J Pharmacol Exp Ther 109:444–452, 1953.
43. Jusko WJ, Lewis GP, Schmitt GW: Ampicillin and hetacillin pharmacokinetics in normal and anephric subjects. Clin Pharmacol Ther 14:90–99, 1973.
44. Kalm O, Kamme C, Bergstrom B, et al: Erythromycin stearate in acute maxillary sinusitis. Scand J Infect Dis 7:209–217, 1975.
45. Kaplan K, Weinstein L: Lincomycin. Pediatr Clin North Am 15:131–137, 1968.
46. Keefer CS: Streptomycin in the treatment of infections. JAMA 132:4–11, 1946.
47. Kirby WM, De Maine JB, Serrill WS: Pharmacokinetics of the cephalosporins in healthy volunteers and uremic patients. Postgrad Med J 47:Suppl:41–46, 1971.
48. Kirby WM, Kind AC: Clinical pharmacology of ampicillin and hetacillin. Ann NY Acad Sci 145:291–297, 1967.
49. Kirby WM, Regamey C: Pharmacokinetics of cefazolin compared with four other cephalosporins. J Infect Dis 128:Suppl:S341–346, 1973.
50. Knudsen ET, Rolinson GN, Sutherland R: Carbenicillin: a new semisynthetic penicillin active against *Pseudomonas pyocyanea*. Br Med J 3:75–78, 1967.
51. Kramer PW, Griffith RS, Campbell RL: Antibiotic penetration of the brain. A comparative study. J Neurosurg 31:295–302, 1969.
52. Kunin CM: A guide to the use of antibiotics in patients with renal disease. A table of recommended doses and factors governing serum levels. Ann Intern Med 67:151–158, 1967.
53. Kunin CM: Antibiotic usage in patients with renal impairment. Hosp Pract Jan:141–149, 1972.
54. Kunin CM: Clinical significance of protein binding of the penicillins. Ann NY Acad Sci 145:282–290, 1967.
55. Kunin CM: The tetracyclines. Pediatr Clin North Am 15:43–53, 1968.
56. Kunin CM, Atuk N: Excretion of cephaloridine and cephalothin in patients with renal impairment. N Engl J Med 274:654–656, 1966.
57. Kunin CM, Brandt D, Wood H: Bacteriologic studies of rifampin, a new semisynthetic antibiotic. J Infect Dis 119:132–137, 1969.
58. Kunin CM, Bugg A: Binding of polymyxin antibiotics to tissues: the major determinant of distribution and persistence in the body. J Infect Dis 124:394–400, 1971.
59. Kunin CM, Finland M: Persistence of antibiotics in blood of patients with acute renal failure. III. Penicillin, streptomycin, erythromycin and kanamycin. J Clin Invest 38:1509–1519, 1959.
60. Kunin CM, Jones WF Jr, Finland M: Enhancement of tetracycline blood levels. N Engl J Med 259:147–156, 1958.
61. Lahikainen EA: Penicillin concentration in middle ear secretion in otitis. Acta Otolaryngol (Stockh) 70:358–362, 1970.
62. Leibowitz BJ, Hakes JL, Cahn MM, et al: Doxycycline blood levels in normal subjects after intravenous and oral administration. Curr Ther Res 14:820–832, 1972.
63. Lester W: Rifampin: A semisynthetic derivative of rifamycin—a prototype for the future. Annu Rev Microbiol 26:85–102, 1972.
64. Linquist JA, Siddiqui JJ, Smith IM: Cephalexin in patients with renal disease. N Engl J Med 283:720–723, 1970.
65. Lundberg C, Malmborg AS, Ivemark BI: Antibiotic concentrations in relation to structural changes in maxillary sinus mucosa following intramuscular or peroral treatment. Scand J Infect Dis 6:187–195, 1974.
66. Mattie H, Goslings WR, Noach EL: Cloxacillin and nafcillin: serum binding and its relationship to antibacterial effect in mice. J Infect Dis 128:170–177, 1973.
67. McCarthy CG, Finland M: Absorption and excretion of four penicillins: penicillin G, penicillin V, phenethicillin, and phenylmercaptomethyl penicillin. N Engl J Med 263:315–326, 1960.
68. McGehee RF, Smith CB, Wilcox C, et al: Comparative studies of antibacterial activity in vitro and absorption and excretion of lincomycin and clinimycin. Am J Med Sci 256:279–292, 1968.
69. McHenry MC, Gavan TL, Gifford RW Jr, et al: Gentamicin dosages for renal insufficiency. Adjustments based on endogenous creatinine clearance and serum creatinine concentration. Ann Intern Med 74:192–197, 1971.

70. McPherson SD Jr, Presley GD, Crawford JR: Aqueous humor assays of subconjunctival antibiotics. Am J Ophthalmol 66:430–435, 1968.
71. Metzger WI, Jenkins CJ Jr, Harris CJ, et al: Laboratory and clinical studies of intramuscular erythromycin. Antibiot Annu 383–386, 1958–1959.
72. Mortimer PR, Mackie DB, Haynes S: Ampicillin levels in human bile in the presence of biliary tract disease. Br Med J 3:88–89, 1969.
73. Neu HC: Antimicrobial activity and human pharmacology of amoxicillin. J Infect Dis 129:Suppl:S123–131, 1974.
74. Orme BM, Cutler RE: The relationship between kanamycin pharmacokinetics: distribution and renal function. Clin Pharmacol Ther 10:543–550, 1969.
75. Parker RH, Schmid FR: Antibacterial activity of synovial fluid during therapy of septic arthritis. Arthritis Rheum 14:96–104, 1971.
76. Pindell MH, Cull KM, Doran KM, et al: Absorption and excretion studies on tetracycline. J Pharmacol Exp Ther 125:287–294, 1959.
77. Pitts RF: Physiology of the Kidney and Body Fluids, ed. 2. Chicago, Year Book Medical Publishers, 1968, p. 131.
77a. Pohjanpelto PEJ, Sarmela TJ, Raines T: Penetration of trimethoprim and sulphamethoxazole into the aqueous humor. Br J Ophthalmol 58:606–608, 1974.
78. Rall DP: Drug entry into brain and cerebro-spinal fluid. In Handbook of Experimental Pharmacology: Concepts in Biochemical Pharmacology, Part I. Edited by Brodie BB, Gillette JR. Springer-Verlag, New York, 1971, pp. 240–248.
79. Ram MD, Watanatittan S: Levels of cefazolin in human bile. J Infect Dis 128:Suppl:S361–363, 1973.
80. Records RE: Intraocular penetration of cephalothin. Am J Ophthalmol 66:436–440, 1968.
81. Reidenberg MM, Shear L, Cohen RV: Elimination of isoniazid in patients with impaired renal function. Am Rev Resp Dis 108:1426–1428, 1973.
82. Ries K, Kaye D: The newer antibiotics. Med Clin North Am 57:1065–1078, 1973.
83. Sabath LD, Postic B, Finland M: Laboratory studies on methicillin. Am J Med Sci 244:484–500, 1962.
84. Sachs J, Geer T, Noell P, et al: Effect of renal function on urinary recovery of orally administered nitrofurantoin. N Engl J Med 278:1032–1035, 1968.
85. Schwartz DE, Ziegler WH: Assay and pharmacokinetics of trimethoprim in man and animals. Postgrad Med J 45:Suppl:32–37, 1969.
86. Sharpstone P: The renal handling of trimethoprim and sulphamethoxazole in man. Postgrad Med J 45:Suppl:38–42, 1969.
87. Siemienski J, Cade R, Kaplan N, Braude AI: A comparison of penicillin blood levels obtained by inhibition of excretion with those obtained by enhancing absorption. Am J Med Sci 235:517–522, 1958.
88. Simon HJ: Streptomycin, kanamycin, neomycin and paromomycin. Pediatr Clin North Am 15:73–83, 1968.
89. Spector R, Lorenzo AV: The effects of salicylate and probenecid on the cerebrospinal fluid transport of penicillin, aminosalicylic acid and iodide. J Pharmacol Exp Ther 188:55–65, 1974.
90. Stamey T: Urinary infections. Baltimore, The Williams & Wilkins Co., 1972, pp. 161–200.
91. Standiford HC, Jordan MC, Kirby WM: Clinical pharmacology of carbenicillin compared with other penicillins. J Infect Dis 122:Suppl:S9–13, 1970.
92. Steigbigel NH, Reed CW, Finland M: Absorption and excretion of five tetracycline analogues in normal young men. Am J Med Sci 255:296–312, 1968.
93. Stratford BC, Dixson S: Serum levels of gentamicin and tobramycin after slow intravenous bolus injection. Lancet 1:378–379, 1974.
94. Suhrland LG, Weisberger AS: Chloramphenicol toxicity in liver and renal disease. Arch Intern Med 112:747–754, 1963.
95. Sutherland R, Croydon EA, Rolinson GN: Flucloxacillin, a new isoxazolyl penicillin, compared with oxacillin, cloxacillin, and dicloxacillin. Br Med J 4:455–460, 1970.
96. Thornhill TS, Levison ME, Johnson WD, et al: In vitro antimicrobial activity and human pharmacology of cephalexin, a new orally absorbed cephalosporin C antibiotic. Appl Microb 17:457–461, 1969.
97. Tuano SB, Brodie JL, Kirby WM: Cephaloridine versus cephalothin: relation of the kidney to blood level differences after parenteral administration. Antimicrob Agents Chemother 101–106, 1966.

98. Tuano SB, Johnson LD, Brodie JL, et al: Comparative blood levels of hetacillin, ampicillin and penicillin G. N Engl J Med 275:635–639, 1966.
99. Venuto RC, Plaut ME: Cephalothin handling in patients undergoing hemodialysis. Antimicrob Agents Chemother 50–52, 1970.
100. Waalkes TP, Denham C, DeVita VT: Pentamidine: clinical pharmacologic correlations in man and mice. Clin Pharmacol Ther 11:505–512, 1970.
101. Wagner JG, Novak E, Patel NC, et al: Absorption, excretion and half-life of clinimycin in normal adult males. Am J Med Sci 256:25–37, 1968.
102. Welling P, Craig W, Amidon G, et al: Pharmacokinetics of trimethoprim and sulfamethoxazole in normal subjects and in patients with renal failure. J Infect Dis 128:Suppl:S556–566, 1973.
103. Whelton A, Sapir DG, Carter GG, et al: Intrarenal distribution of ampicillin in the normal and diseased human kidney. J Infect Dis 125:466–470, 1972.
104. Zintel HA, Flippin H, Nichols A, et al: Studies on streptomycin in man, absorption, distribution, excretion and toxicity. Am J Med Sci 210:421–430, 1945.

CHAPTER 6

HARMFUL REACTIONS, INCOMPATIBILITIES, AND INTERACTIONS OF ANTIMICROBIAL DRUGS

Antimicrobials can injure the patient through direct toxicity, hypersensitivity, rapid lysis of the infectious agent, and disturbance in normal microbial flora.

DIRECT TOXICITY

Blood

The mechanisms of blood cell injury by chloramphenicol, amphotericin B, trimethoprim, and 5–fluorocytosine are probably similar to those responsible for their antimicrobial activity (Table 6–1). Small concentrations of chloramphenicol inhibit protein synthesis in mammalian cells by impairing mitochondrial protein synthesis, but not protein synthesis on ribosomes in the cytoplasm.[85] This selective effect on mitochondrial protein synthesis is probably related to the fact that ribosomes of mammalian mitochondria strongly resemble in behavior the 70S ribosomes found in bacteria and that the major subunits of mitochondrial ribosomes are of the bacterial or 50S type. The inhibition of mitochondrial protein synthesis by chloramphenicol would be expected to impair the production of structural proteins. Electron micrographs of mitochondria in the marrow cells of patients receiving chloramphenicol show a change in ultrastructural organization characterized by an increase in density of the mitochondrial matrix.[130] All cell types within the marrow are susceptible to the change, and a striking correlation is said to exist between the number of cells with

TABLE 6–1. *Direct Toxicity of Antimicrobial Drugs: Blood*

DRUG	PROBABLE MECHANISM OF TOXICITY	CHIEF CLINICAL SIGNS
Chloramphenicol	Inhibition of mitochondrial protein synthesis Change in genetic structure of stem cells	Reversible leukopenia, anemia, and thrombocytopenia Fatal aplastic anemia
Chloramphenicol, sulfonamides, nitrofurantoin, and primaquine	G6PD deficiency	Hemolytic anemia
Amphotericin B	Erythrocyte membrane injury	Reversible normocytic, normochromic anemia
Trimethoprim	Folate deficiency	Leukopenia, thrombocytopenia, and megaloblastic anemia
Carbenicillin	Decreased sensitivity of platelets to aggregation by ADP	Excessive surgical bleeding
5-Fluorocytosine	Abnormal nucleic acid synthesis only in renal insufficiency	Aplastic anemia and leukopenia

mitochondrial injury and the serum level of chloramphenicol. Changes are first noticed at serum levels of 11 μg/ml and become extensive at about 30 μg/ml. When the drug is discontinued, however, the ultrastructural changes in mitochondria are no longer detectable. These observations have been used to explain reversible bone marrow suppression from chloramphenicol.[130]

Many, if not all, patients given chloramphenicol will eventually sustain such marrow suppression. A few weeks after the drug is started, the serum iron level rises and the blood hemoglobin level falls as less iron is used for hemoglobin synthesis. At the same time reticulocytes and normoblasts decrease, and cytoplasmic vacuolation appears in early erythroid forms and granulocyte precursors. Platelet counts may also drop. Since these abnormalities are a function of chloramphenicol concentration and appear regularly with levels of 25 μg/ml or higher, they are more likely to occur in patients with liver disease who are less able to inactivate the drug. Once chloramphenicol is stopped, the blood picture returns to normal in two weeks. Although tetracycline can also inhibit protein synthesis, it does not affect mitochondrial protein synthesis and does not produce clinical bone marrow suppression, possibly because of its avidity for metal cations, such as calcium, which could prevent accumulation of the drug in marrow cells.[130]

Chloramphenicol also produces a rare form of irreversible and fatal aplastic anemia that seems to have a different pathogenesis than the reversible form of marrow suppression, and is not related to the amount or length of exposure to chloramphenicol. In the benign form of marrow suppression, chloramphenicol interferes with maturation and division of differentiated cells, while in malignant marrow aplasia and pancytopenia the drug apparently prevents differentiation of stem cells by changing their genetic structure. It is reported that chloramphenicol can cause vacuolization of chromosomes, a change that could evolve into irreversible changes in stem cells.[92] Obscure constitutional and regional predispositions have been proposed to explain differences in the incidence of fatal pancytopenia from chloramphenicol. The incidence seems higher in South America and Australia than in Israel or West Germany. Its occurrence in identical twins raises the question of genetic predisposition.[94]

While genetic factors have only been suspected in chloramphenicol-induced aplastic anemia, they have been well established in the hemolytic anemias caused by chloramphenicol in patients with deficiencies in erythrocyte glucose-6-phosphate dehydrogenase (G6PD).[11] This type of hemolysis is seen only in subjects with less than 30 per cent of the normal amount of G6PD in their red blood cells. The gene determining the structure of G6PD is carried on the X chromosome and therefore is sex-linked. Among Caucasians, the Mediterranean type of abnormal G6PD is the most common, reaching an incidence of 50 per cent among Kurdish Jews. Chloramphenicol may bring about hemolytic episodes in the Mediterranean type, but not the milder A type of deficiency. The unstable A type of G6PD is the commonest form in American Negroes. Eleven per cent of American Negro males are affected, and their red blood cells contain only 5 to 15 per cent of the normal amount of enzyme activity. The antimalarial primaquine will induce hemolysis in both types. Nitrofuran derivatives and sulfonamides can also be responsible for hemolytic anemia in patients with G6PD-deficient red blood cells. The exact mechanism of red blood cell hemolysis is not known, but cells deficient in G6PD activity cannot reduce NADP (nicotinamide adenine dinucleotide phosphate) to NADPH at a normal rate. Since NADPH is a cofactor for glutathione reductase, G6PD-deficient cells have inadequate concentrations of glutathione to maintain the integrity of the erythrocyte membrane. In the A type of G6PD deficiency, the hemolysis subsides upon the appearance of new red blood cells because their levels of G6PD are close to normal, and the offending drug may be continued without preventing recovery from anemia.[33]

Anemia is also a constant feature of treatment with amphotericin B, and seems to be caused by an injury to the erythrocyte membrane with loss of potassium and other essential intracellular constituents[16, 27] (Fig. 6-1). Red blood cells rapidly take up the drug, which is probably bound to cholesterol in the cell membrane as in yeasts. This uptake is diminished by plasma, possibly by competition for binding of amphotericin by plasma sterols. During treatment with amphotericin B the average concentration in plasma of 1 μg/ml is too low to injure red blood cells, but at the site of infusion into the vein the concentration is often 75 to 200 μg/ml and the drug would be rapidly taken up by red blood cells. It could then produce enough red blood cell injury during long-term therapy to account for part

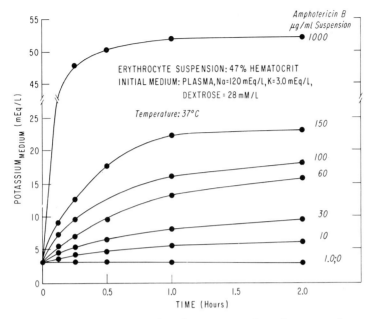

Figure 6–1. Effect of concentration of amphotericin B on loss of potassium from erythrocytes. (From Butler WT, Cotlove E: Increased permeability of human erythrocytes induced by amphotericin B. J Infect Dis *123*:343. © 1971 by the University of Chicago Press.)

of the anemia without producing generalized changes in red blood cells that would be reflected in survival or fragility assays. Since the normocytic anemia is not accompanied by reticulocytosis, hypochromia, or erythroid hyperplasia, it has also been suggested that amphotericin suppresses red blood cell production. The azotemia during amphotericin B treatment may also be a factor in producing anemia.

The other synthetic antifungal drug in common use, 5-fluorocytosine (5FC), does not cause anemia or other blood disorders except in renal failure. Then it can produce marrow suppression ranging from pancytopenia to mild leukopenia.[12] The mechanism of marrow toxicity is unknown, but may be inferred from the mode of action against yeasts. As noted in Chapter 2, 5FC is converted to 5-fluorouracil (5FU) in yeast cells but not in mammalian cells, which lack cytosine deaminase. In man the intestinal flora are probably responsible for converting 5FC to 5FU.

Bone marrow suppression by trimethoprim is probably a manifestation of folate deficiency. Although dihydrofolic reductase in man is more resistant to inhibition by trimethoprim than the bacterial enzyme, the drug can interfere with human folate metabolism if given in excessive doses and for long periods.[62] Leukopenia, anemia, and thrombocytopenia can be expected in a few patients if the dose of trimethoprim is larger than 200 mg daily, if high levels result from impaired renal excretion, or if the drug is used in conjunction with other antimetabolites that suppress the marrow.[58, 127] The hematologic changes are usually reversible if folinic acid is

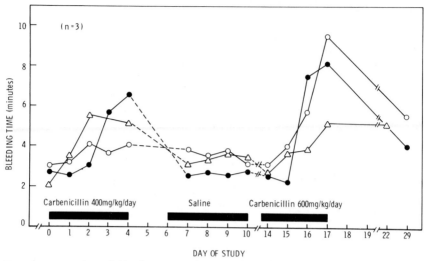

Figure 6–2. Prolonged bleeding times during carbenicillin administration. (From Brown CH, et al: The hemostatic defect produced by carbenicillin. N Engl J Med 291:266, 1974.)

given, or if the drug is stopped. Older patients receiving diuretics and renal transplant patients treated with azathioprine seem especially vulnerable to hematologic depression by trimethoprim-sulfamethoxazole. Because the two antimicrobials are generally used together, the importance of trimethoprim alone in causing blood changes is not always clear, but there is no question that trimethoprim can produce folate deficiency leading to hematologic changes.

In contrast to these drugs, whose toxic effects on blood elements can be related to their antimicrobial action, a serious platelet injury is caused by carbenicillin and other penicillins through unknown mechanisms. When carbenicillin is given in doses recommended for treatment of infection, all recipients develop defective platelet function within 12 to 24 hours.[19] The drug, or a metabolite, appears to impair the function of platelets by decreasing their sensitivity to aggregation by adenosine diphosphate (ADP). Since ADP is the physiologic agent responsible for aggregation into platelet plugs that repair blood vessels, it is not surprising that carbenicillin frequently causes prolonged bleeding and that it appears to be responsible for bleeding problems after surgery[88] (Fig. 6–2).

A number of other antibiotics are anticoagulants but only when used in greater concentration than can be attained in the blood.[17] Oxytetracycline, for example, is almost as good an anticoagulant as sodium citrate. Since the aminoglycosides and penicillin prevent blood coagulation in concentrations of 20 to 30 mg/ml, they could reduce clotting at the site of intramuscular injection. Like its neurotoxicity, the anticoagulant effect of streptomycin can be reversed with calcium. Table 6–1 summarizes the direct toxic effects of antimicrobial drugs on the blood.

Kidney

The antibiotics that are directly toxic to the kidney are also those that are poorly absorbed from the gut. These are the aminoglycosides, polymyxins, polyenes, and cephaloridine. The polymyxins and polyenes share two other properties, tissue binding and membrane injury, which might be factors in their nephrotoxicity. Otherwise, the various nephrotoxic drugs are too dissimilar chemically and functionally to operate through a common mechanism of renal injury, and each must be considered individually (Table 6–2).

Amphotericin B, the only polyene given systemically, reduces renal blood flow and creatinine clearance and causes distal tubular acidosis (without the loss of amino acids, bicarbonate, or glucose in the urine seen in proximal tubular acidosis).[23, 38] Amphotericin seems to produce a permeability defect that allows the tubular cells to leak potassium and become permeable to hydrogen ions (Fig. 6–3). Hydrogen ions can then pass from the tubular urine into the cells. Concentrating ability is also impaired. The overall picture of amphotericin toxicity to the kidney is one of azotemia, acidosis, hypokalemia, and polyuria. These disturbances develop slowly during chronic treatment in association with vacuolization of tubular cells and calcium deposition in tubules and interstitium. All functional abnormalities are reversible in most cases, but a total dose of over 5.0 gm of amphotericin may cause permanent renal failure and severe nephrocalcinosis.[26] The most dangerous immediate problem is hypokalemia, which requires early potassium replacement. Daily supplements of 100 mEq of potassium are often needed after even small doses of amphotericin. Prevention of hypokalemia does not avert renal tubular acidosis, but fortunately systemic acidosis is rare.[38, 89] The syndrome is usually limited to an elevation of minimum urinary pH and a depression of titratable acid excretion

TABLE 6–2.   *Direct Toxicity of Antimicrobial Drugs: Kidney*

DRUG	PROBABLE MECHANISM OF TOXICITY	CHIEF CLINICAL SIGNS
Amphotericin B	Reduced renal flow and distal tubular permeability defect	Hypokalemia, tubular acidosis, and nephrocalcinosis
Neomycin, kanamycin, and gentamicin	Injury to proximal tubules	Cylinduria, albuminuria, and azotemia
Polymyxin B and colistin	Tubular damage	Azotemia
Cephaloridine	Proximal tubular damage	Azotemia
Stale tetracycline	Proximal tubular damage	Fanconi syndrome
Demethylchlor-tetracycline	Inhibition of antidiuretic hormone	Nephrogenic diabetes insipidus

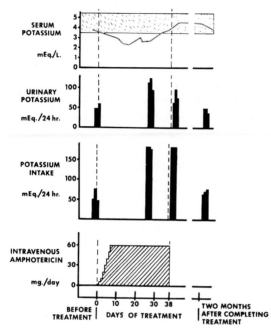

Figure 6–3. The effects of amphotericin B treatment on serum potassium level and the rate of urinary excretion of potassium. (From Douglas JB, Healy JK: Nephrotoxic effects of amphotericin B, including renal tubular acidosis. Am J Med 46:157, 1969.)

in response to acid loading with ammonium chloride. Aside from providing potassium supplements, the main precaution is to discontinue the drug temporarily if the blood urea nitrogen reaches 40 mg per 100 ml.

The aminoglycosides also injure renal tubules. The severest renal injury is caused by neomycin, followed in order of nephrotoxicity by kanamycin, gentamicin, and spectinomycin. Streptomycin, on the other hand, is probably not nephrotoxic in the usual clinical dosages. Neomycin damages tubules severely after daily intramuscular doses of 1.0 gm for more than two weeks. All the proximal convoluted tubules may show extensive necrosis of the epithelium with sloughing of these cells into the tubular lumen. Swelling and vacuolization are also prominent (Fig. 6–4). The glomeruli, on the other hand, are spared. The most consistent early clinical evidence of neomycin renal injury is the presence of albumin and fine granular casts in the urine. Azotemia develops later and may be reversible if the drug is stopped. Kanamycin and gentamicin can also cause reversible albuminuria, casts, and azotemia, but severe anatomic changes like those found with neomycin are unusual in patients. The nephrotoxicity of both drugs increases with dose, age, and the presence of underlying kidney disease, but occasionally patients with no sign of kidney disease may develop severe renal insufficiency on usual doses. The incidence of abnormal kidney function after gentamicin can be as high as 45 per cent in patients with normal function before treatment.[128] Equivalent doses of gentamicin in experimental animals produce ultrastructural changes in the lysosomes of convoluted tubular cells, but morphologic evidence of such injury in patients has not been reported.[67]

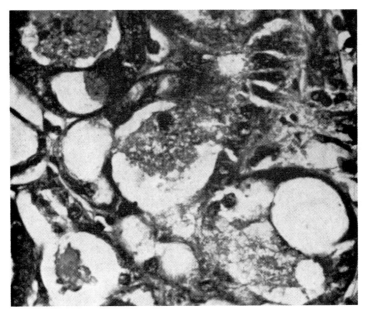

Figure 6–4. Necrosis and vacuolation of tubular epithelium after neomycin therapy. (From Powell LW, Hooker JW: Neomycin nephropathy. JAMA 160:560, 1956.)

The polymyxins can also injure the epithelium of renal convoluted tubules. All patients receiving either polymyxin B or E (colistin) in ordinary doses should be monitored carefully for diminished urine output and rising blood urea nitrogen or creatinine because serious tubular injury may occur regardless of dose or duration of therapy. Deterioration of renal function may be arrested by discontinuing the polymyxins, and nephrotoxicity is often reversible, but the azotemia may progress for several weeks after the drug has been stopped. Very high, sustained plasma levels of polymyxins consistently produce acute renal failure after excessive doses in patients with normal kidneys and after ordinary doses in patients with underlying renal failure.[101] About 20 per cent of the patients receiving colistin have suffered renal damage, and about 1.9 per cent develop acute tubular necrosis. For unknown reasons, cephalothin appears to increase the nephrotoxic potential of colistin[66] and gentamicin.[14]

Among cephalosporins, celphaloridine stands out as the most nephrotoxic. It has caused acute proximal tubular necrosis in both patients and animals, and the nephrotoxicity is related to the dose.[116] Daily doses should be kept below 4.0 gm in adults to avoid renal damage.[9] Since cefazolin has not been reported to cause kidney injury and since it can also be injected intramuscularly, there is no reason to risk tubular injury from cephaloridine.

Two unusual reversible forms of tubular dysfunction are caused by the tetracyclines. Demethylchlortetracycline can produce nephrogenic diabetes insipidus, and outdated ("stale") tetracycline can induce the Fanconi syndrome. Although full-blown diabetes insipidus with polyuria, polydipsia, and weakness is rarely observed, about one-third of the patients taking demethylchlortetracycline for acne are said to have renal concentrating defects.[117] The incidence and severity of the concentrating defect increase in proportion to the dose and seem to be caused by the impaired response of the collecting tubules to the antidiuretic hormone (ADH). It is postulated that ADH stimulates water flow across the collecting duct by activating adenylcyclase to produce cyclic AMP and that cyclic AMP increases transepithelial water permeability. Demethylchlortetracycline probably inhibits both the production and the action of cyclic AMP. This renal effect of demethylchlortetracycline has been used to advantage for treating water retention in patients with inappropriate secretion of ADH.[33a]

The Fanconi syndrome is seen in patients taking ordinary tetracycline that has deteriorated from storage in warm, moist conditions so that the granular powder changes to a gummy material or a hard black plug. The toxic degradation products appear to be epitetracycline, epianhydrotetracycline, and anhydrotetracycline. These cause a clinical picture resembling diabetes mellitus with acidosis, nausea, vomiting, proteinuria, glycosuria, and aminoaciduria. Recovery occurs in about one month after the toxic tetracycline ingestion has been stopped.[44]

A more common effect of tetracyclines on the kidneys is seen when there is pre-existing renal failure. Azotemia is aggravated by the anticatabolic effect of the tetracyclines. They inhibit protein synthesis by preventing the transfer of amino acids from aminoacyl-tRNA. These amino acids then undergo deamination, and the freed amino groups are converted to excess urea in the liver. Since renal function is not disturbed, the rise in blood urea is not accompanied by elevated creatinine levels. The tetracyclines may provoke uremic vomiting, however, and the loss of fluid and electrolytes leads to rapid deterioration of renal function. Since doxycycline does not aggravate uremia, it is the one tetracycline that can be given safely to patients in renal failure. Table 6–2 summarizes the direct toxic effects of antimicrobial drugs on the kidney.

Nervous System

Deafness, vestibular injury, neuromuscular paralysis, and encephalopathy are the main toxic effects of antibiotics on the nervous system. The aminoglycosides cause deafness by injuring the organ of Corti. Neomycin, the most potent cause of deafness, damages primarily the inner hair cells of the organ of Corti in the human ear[43] (Fig. 6–5), and deafness may occur from topical as well as parenteral therapy.[64] Kanamycin is less toxic than neomycin but more so than streptomycin, dihydrostreptomycin, or gentamicin. Kanamycin causes deafness by damaging the outer hair cells and the supporting cells of the organ of Corti[87] (Fig. 6–6). It also causes vestibular damage, perhaps by central injury, since the peripheral vestibular apparatus may be histologically normal when there is no response to massive cold caloric testing. There is experimental evidence

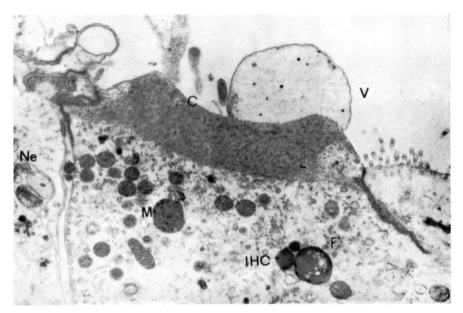

Figure 6–5. Neomycin injury to inner ear is illustrated in electron micrograph of the organ of Corti. The outer membrane of the cell surface of inner hair cell (IHC) forms large vesicles (V) containing cellular debris. Swollen mitochondria (M) and fatty droplets (F) in apical zone are also present. Nerves (Ne) are visible near cuticle (C). (From Friedmann I, Dadswell JV, Bird ES: Electron-microscope studies of the neuro-epithelium of the inner ear in guinea-pigs treated with neomycin. J Pathol Bacteriol 92:418, 1966.)

suggesting that high levels of kanamycin in the endolymph of the inner ear may be responsible for its ototoxicity.[59] By inhibiting adenosinetriphosphatase (ATPase) in the stria vascularis of the cochlea, kanamycin blocks the energy source required for its own removal from the cochlea and thereby causes its own accumulation there. The earliest effect of kanamycin on the ear is a subtle loss of high-frequency tones. This loss can be picked up only by audiometry because conversational tones are under 2000 cycles per second. Since the outer hair cells can probably recover at this stage, regular audiometric examination is necessary to prevent deafness in patients receiving kanamycin. This is especially important in older patients and in others with impaired renal function because impaired excretion causes high levels of the drug in the blood that would be reflected in the endolymph of the organ of Corti. Even with normal renal function, periodic audiometry is important because of the marked biological variation in susceptibility to the ototoxic effects of antibiotics. The overall incidence of clinically apparent ototoxicity from kanamycin is 5 per cent.

Whereas neomycin and kanamycin cause selective injury to hair cells, streptomycin selectively injures the sensory cells of the vestibular system. Dihydrostreptomycin resembles the others in its predilection for the organ of Corti.[71] The dihydrostreptomycin effect has a long latent period between the cessation of the drug and the onset of deafness. While some patients also suffer loss of vestibular function after dihydrostreptomycin, vestibular

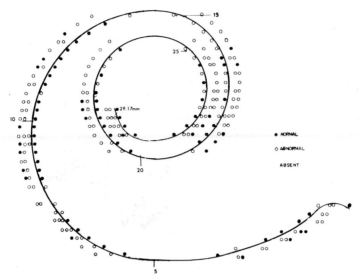

Figure 6–6. Graphic reconstruction of the right human cochlea showing the severe outer hair cell destruction from kanamycin with relative sparing of the inner hair cells. (From Ward PH, et al: The ototoxicity of kanamycin. Laryngoscope 75:5, 1965.)

damage is more marked after streptomycin treatment. Very small doses of streptomycin may cause vertigo while the patient is walking, as well as a reduced caloric response in susceptible patients; but if the dose is not over 1 gm per day, the effect usually appears only after prolonged treatment. With doses of 2 gm daily, vestibular symptoms usually appear in three to four weeks. In addition to vertigo, streptomycin poisoning causes ataxia, but fortunately the patient can adapt eventually to vestibular damage by visual clues and deep proprioceptive sensation. Adaptation begins in a few months, and full recovery may take over a year. In a few patients, streptomycin can also cause high-frequency hearing impairment outside the conversational range after one week. This can be detected only by audiometric examination. Patients may also experience high-pitched tinnitus that subsides in less than two weeks after the drug is stopped. Hearing loss in the conversational range may appear later, but complete deafness is rare. Infants of mothers treated with streptomycin can develop abnormal caloric reactions and minor hearing loss. As a general rule streptomycin should be used with extreme caution in pregnancy, in older patients who have trouble adapting to vestibular damage, and in patients who already have hearing difficulty. The incidence of ototoxicity from streptomycin is 3.6 per cent.[63]

Although gentamicin also affects principally the vestibular system, it can cause deafness. Experimentally, the most severe injury is found in the vestibular sensory cells but higher doses damage the outer hair cells of the cochlea[82] as well. The incidence of vestibular toxicity from gentamicin varies from 2.3 to 10 per cent, rising with age and impaired renal function.[3,98] Unlike the ototoxic effect of streptomycin or kanamycin, damage to the ear from gentamicin occurs more often in one ear than in both.[91] About 30 per cent of the patients who develop vestibular impairment also have concomitant high-tone hearing loss. The main complaint is transient dizziness.

Aside from the aminoglycosides, only minocycline has been a prominent cause of vestibular reactions.[129] In the United States, a number of patients receiving minocycline for meningococcal prophylaxis developed dizziness, vertigo, nausea, and vomiting after a total dose of only 400 mg.[2] Studies in England and Brazil using minocycline processed in those countries also reported vestibular reactions to the antibiotic, but their incidence was much lower than in the United States.[2,86,96] The mechanism of vestibular side effects is unknown.

The aminoglycosides are a major cause of neuromuscular blockade, sharing this toxicity with colistin and polymyxin B. The major catastrophe from this toxicity is respiratory arrest, which has been observed after intraperitoneal neomycin sulfate, kanamycin sulfate, and streptomycin sulfate; intrapleural neomycin sulfate; and intravenous kanamycin sulfate, streptomycin sulfate, and gentamicin sulfate.[125] On the other hand, all cases of respiratory paralysis after colistin have followed intramuscular injection,[80] while polymyxin B has caused apnea after either intramuscular or intravenous injection. Two types of mechanisms appear responsible for the blockade at the myoneural end-plate. The aminoglycosides produce a competitive blockade in which the drug probably competes with acetylcholine for receptor sites so that the end-plate is not depolarized and muscle fibers cannot contract. This form of competitive blockade is also produced by d-tubocurarine, the purified constituent of curare, and is reversed by anticholinesterase compounds, such as neostigmine. Patients who develop respiratory paralysis from aminoglycosides should receive 0.25 mg neostigmine intravenously every 30 minutes. This small dose of neostigmine can bring about dramatic improvement with only mild muscarinic effects that can be controlled with atropine.[103]

The second type of blockade is produced by colistin and polymyxin B. It is neostigmine-resistant and noncompetitive.[20] Since the main effect of these two antibiotics is a prolonged period of depolarization associated with local calcium depletion, the paralysis is treated by intravenous injection of 5.0 gm of calcium gluconate.[131]

A number of cases of respiratory paralysis associated with antibiotics have been seen during or just after anesthesia, but the aminoglycosides and polymyxins can produce neuromuscular paralysis in nonsurgical, nonanesthetized patients as well.[80] The neurotoxicity is dose-related, and the problem of blockade is therefore most likely when the drug is given into the peritoneum where the absorptive surface is so great that high levels develop rapidly, when the patient is uremic, and when there is an accidental overdosage.

Among the antibiotics, penicillin is the principal cause of brain damage. It consistently produces seizures when topically applied to the cerebral cortex in high concentrations and requires an intact lactam ring because its convulsive effect is abolished with penicillinase.[52] Experimentally, it produces an epileptic focus characterized by a recurring, isolated high-voltage negative wave (the interictal spike of the electroencephalograph), thought to result from a lowering of the threshold for impulse initiation.[7] Seizures resulting from penicillin were first observed after intraventricular, intracisternal, or intrathecal administration of the drug in doses ranging from 40,000 to 50,000 units for the treatment of meningitis and general paresis, and for prophylaxis after neurosurgery.

More recently, seizures have occurred after the intravenous administration of over 25 million units of penicillin to middle-aged or elderly patients with renal insufficiency, or during cardiopulmonary bypass.[13, 113] The brain is ordinarily protected by the blood-brain barrier from such massive doses of penicillin, but in renal insufficiency high blood levels are attained by continuous infusion, thereby breaching the barrier and producing a progressive rise in spinal fluid concentration as the drug accumulates faster than it can be removed. The first clinical sign of penicillin brain injury after massive intravenous therapy in uremia is a decrease in the level of consciousness eight hours after the start of treatment. Soon afterward, myoclonic jerks appear in the face, pectoral girdle, and extremities. Status epilepticus may alternate with the focal seizures.[13]

Seizures during cardiopulmonary bypass are blamed on increased permeability of the blood-brain barrier. When 50 million units of penicillin are given intravenously before, during, and after the operation to prevent postsurgical endocarditis, the patient may never regain consciousness after anesthesia and may die of continuous generalized seizures[113] (Fig. 6–7). As a result of these catastrophes, massive penicillin prophylaxis has been discontinued in heart surgery and the drug is used with caution in uremia. Other penicillin and cephalosporin drugs can also induce seizures in uremia. Although remarkably nontoxic to the brain of patients receiving massive doses, carbenicillin has produced seizures in the presence of severe azotemia and oliguria.[57]

Occasional reports of toxic brain disorders have also been reported with other antimicrobials. Large doses of nalidixic acid can produce a wide spectrum of reversible encephalopathic syndromes ranging from syncope, seizures, or acute psychoses in adults to intracranial hypertension in infants.[28, 41, 42] Benign intracranial hypertension has also occurred after tetracycline treatment. Bulging of the anterior fontanelles in infants, and headache, photophobia, and papilledema in older children or adults all clear up when the tetracycline is stopped.[65, 84] One report on "chloramphenicol encephalopathy" describes acute delirium during the chloramphenicol treatment of some cases with multiple myeloma and one with carcinoma of the sigmoid.[79] The appearance of chloramphenicol-associated encephalopathy after oral, but not after parenteral medication at the same dosage, suggested that abnormal liver function, related to high portal drug concentration, might be responsible.

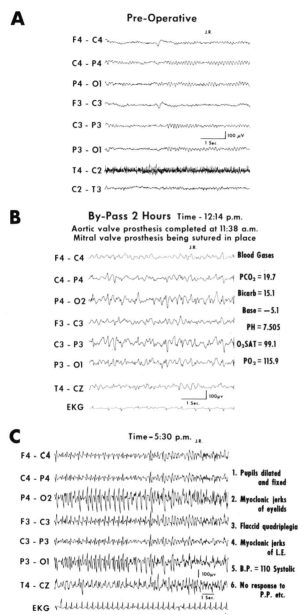

Figure 6–7. Induction of seizures by penicillin during cardiopulmonary bypass. Before, during, and after the bypass procedure the patient received 50,000,000 units of sodium crystalline penicillin. Electroencephalograms taken before the operation are shown in *A*. In *B*, bioccipital epileptiform sharp waves first appear with the patient in bypass for two hours. In *C*, generalized seizure activity is shown early in the postoperative period when he was in status epilepticus. (From Seamans KB, Gloor P, Dobell ARC: Penicillin-induced seizures during cardiopulmonary bypass. N Engl J Med 278:863, 1968.)

Optic neuritis, which may lead to permanent blindness, is another rare effect of chloramphenicol. It is seen primarily in children being given prolonged treatment for cystic fibrosis. They recover at least partial vision, however, after the chloramphenicol is stopped and treatment with large doses of B-complex vitamins is instituted. Chloroquine produces another form of visual disturbance, but only after prolonged therapy of months or years for certain noninfectious conditions. The chloroquine visual disturbance is related to a peculiar irreversible retinopathy with macular pigmentation, retinal artery constriction, and loss of central visual activity.

Isoniazid may cause optic neuritis and encephalopathy, but peripheral neuritis is its chief form of neurotoxicity. Although slow acetylators are more likely to accumulate isoniazid and develop peripheral neuritis, the problem can be prevented in all patients by giving 100 mg pyridoxine daily.[69] Two other antituberculosis drugs, ethambutol and cycloserine, are also neurotoxic. Ethambutol causes reversible optic atrophy, and cycloserine causes encephalopathy. Symptoms of cycloserine encephalopathy appear within the first two weeks of treatment and consist of dysarthria, vertigo, confusion, psychotic states, paresis, and convulsions. The convulsions may be prevented by giving 100 mg pyridoxine daily. While cy-

TABLE 6–3.   *Direct Toxicity of Antimicrobial Drugs: Nervous System*

DRUG	PROBABLE MECHANISM OF TOXICITY	CHIEF CLINICAL SIGNS
Neomycin and kanamycin	Injury to inner hair cells of organ of Corti	Deafness
Streptomycin and gentamicin	Injury to sensory cells of vestibular system	Upright vertigo and ataxia
Aminoglycosides	Competitive neuromuscular blockade	Respiratory arrest
Polymyxin B and colistin	Noncompetitive neuromuscular blockade	Respiratory arrest
Penicillins and cephalosporins	Epileptogenic stimulation	Convulsive seizures
Nalidixic acid	Unknown	Reversible seizures, psychoses, and acute intracranial hypertension in infants
Tetracycline	Unknown	Acute intracranial hypertension
Chloramphenicol	Unknown (vitamin B deficiency?)	Optic neuritis, encephalopathy
Isoniazid	Pyridoxine deficiency	Peripheral neuritis, optic atrophy, and encephalopathy
Ethambutol	Unknown	Optic atrophy
Cycloserine	Pyridoxine deficiency (?)	Convulsions, dysarthria, vertigo, and psychoses
Nitrofurantoin	Hydantoin effect	Polyneuritis

closerine is rarely used for tuberculosis, it is regarded as an important substitute for sulfonamides in nocardiosis.

Among the antimicrobial agents, nitrofurantoin is probably the most potent cause of peripheral neuritis.[105] This toxicity may be related to its hydantoin component, since prolonged treatment with high doses of other hydantoins produces peripheral neuropathy. Electromyographic signs of denervation of distal muscles develop in about two-thirds of nitro-furantoin-treated patients with normal renal function, and these electro-myographic changes last for months even though significant symptoms of neuritis are absent in most.[81] The danger of peripheral neuritis exists mainly in patients with renal failure. They may suffer a severe and even fatal progressive polyneuritis, which may appear a few days after treatment or be delayed. Disintegration of the peripheral nerves and nerve roots, and sarcolemmic proliferation with muscle atrophy occur. Limb wastage and depressed reflexes may persist for many months after sensory changes resolve.[39, 93] Table 6–3 summarizes the direct toxic effects of antimicrobial drugs on the nervous system.

Liver

Direct toxicity is seldom a cause of serious liver damage by antimicro-bial agents. The antituberculosis drugs rifampin, isoniazid, and pyra-zinamide all seem to cause some liver injury, but pyrazinamide is rarely used and the other two usually produce only mild changes (Table 6–4). In one series, an oral dose of 600 mg of rifampin raised the serum bilirubin transiently in nearly all subjects, whether or not liver function had been normal initially.[1] Continuous treatment with daily doses of rifam-pin plus isoniazid (600 mg each) also caused an elevation in serum bilirubin

TABLE 6–4. *Direct Toxicity of Antimicrobial Drugs*

SITE	DRUG	PROBABLE MECHANISM OF TOXICITY	CHIEF CLINICAL SIGNS
Liver	Rifampin	Degeneration of liver cells	Jaundice
	Tetracycline	Fatty metamorphosis	Liver failure in late preg-nancy
Bowel	Neomycin	Villous shortening, cellular infiltration, and crypt-cell damage	Malabsorption and steator-rhea
	Clindamycin Lincomycin	Pseudomembranous procto-sigmoiditis	Diarrhea and abdominal cramps
Skin	Nalidixic acid	Phototoxicity	Sunburn, bullae
	Chlortetracycline and demethyl-chlortetracycline	Phototoxicity	Sunburn, onycholysis
Teeth	Tetracyclines	Localization in developing teeth	Discoloration of teeth and hand defects

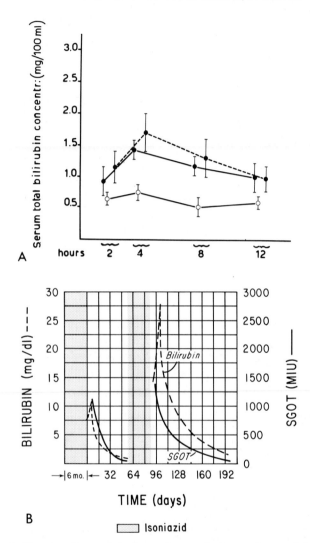

Figure 6–8. *A,* Elevation of serum bilirubin in six normal subjects after 1 oral dose of 600 mg rifampin alone or of isoniazid (600 mg) combined with rifampin (600 mg) (●– – – –●). One oral dose of 600 mg isoniazid alone (O———O) did not raise the serum bilirubin above normal. (From Acocella G, et al: Kinetics of rifampicin and isoniazid administered alone and in combination to normal subjects and patients with liver disease. Gut *13*:49, 1972.)

B, Clinical course of a patient with isoniazid hepatitis is reflected in bilirubin and SGOT levels. By chance the patient was rechallenged with the drug and had a second attack, as shown by the sets of curves on the right. (From Maddrey WC, Boitnott JK: Hepatitis induced by isoniazid and methyldopa. Hosp Pract *10*:122, 1975.)

that returned almost to normal within one week (Fig. 6–8*A*). Since isoniazid alone did not raise the serum bilirubin, rifampin was blamed.[1] Rifampin hepatitis begins within three weeks after start of treatment, and the most severe cases are those with the earliest onset.[70] Biopsies show widespread liver cell degeneration and acidophilic bodies without much inflammation.

The incidence of clinical jaundice in patients given isoniazid and rifampin together may reach 5 to 10 per cent[70] or go higher if the patients have severe alcoholic liver disease. The real danger of rifampin to the liver is still uncertain and variable, but the overall picture from numerous reports suggests that transient mild hyperbilirubinemia is the rule, that combination with isoniazid might increase the possibility of liver injury, and that serious jaundice is probably limited to those with alcoholic hepatic injury.

The risks of developing liver disease from isoniazid alone are very small, varying from 0 to 10 cases per 1000 patients on isoniazid per year.[21] About 12 per cent of isoniazid recipients develop reversible SGOT elevations higher than 100 units/ml (upper limits of normal, 40) (Fig. 6–8B). Isoniazid liver disease does not occur in children and its incidence rises with age. Since its pathology does not differ from that of viral hepatitis, the validity of isoniazid hepatitis as a diagnostic entity has sometimes been doubted. Such doubts have been reinforced by the fact that it cannot be reproduced in animals, is not dose dependent, and has no identifiable predisposing factors. In fact, the consensus is that isoniazid does not cause direct toxic liver injury and that isoniazid hepatitis is an expression of delayed hypersensitivity.[21, 83]

Aside from the antituberculosis drugs, tetracycline is the only antimicrobial seriously implicated as a cause of liver injury. Most cases of severe tetracycline hepatitis have been women given relatively high doses of intravenous tetracycline in late pregnancy for the treatment of pyelonephritis.[112] The striking disorder in fatal cases is a large soft yellow liver with a fine-droplet fatty metamorphosis involving all portions of the lobules but without necrosis, inflammation, or biliary obstruction. Acute pancreatitis may also occur. This condition resembles the acute obstetric fatty metamorphosis that develops without tetracycline, and this antibiotic seems to enhance susceptibility to the disorder.

It is important to keep in mind that a few antibiotics cause abnormalities in liver function tests due to technical factors rather than liver disease. False elevations of SGOT can be induced by para-aminosalicylic acid and erythromycin estolate when the enzyme is assayed by colorimetric methods in the automatic multichannel analyzer. When a patient receiving these drugs has a high level of SGOT, additional tests of liver function should be made before it is assumed that the increase is due to liver damage.[46, 109]

Gastrointestinal Tract

Most antibiotics give rise to gastrointestinal irritability in some patients, but only neomycin, lincomycin, and clindamycin cause severe damage with characteristic morphologic and functional changes in the bowel (Table 6–4). Oral neomycin in doses of 3 to 12 gm daily produces malabsorption of fat, protein, and carbohydrates (Fig. 6–9). Within one week oral neomycin causes striking villous shortening, round cell infiltration in the

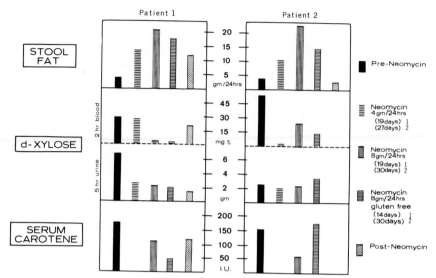

Figure 6–9. Neomycin-induced malabsorption and steatorrhea. Normal values: Stool fat = <7 gm/24 hr; D-xylose in urine = >4 gm/5 hr; D-xylose in blood = >20 mg/100 ml; serum carotene = 100 to 300 IU. (From Rogers AI, et al: Neomycin-induced steatorrhea. JAMA *197*:186, 1966.)

upper small bowel, and crypt-cell damage that resembles the mitochondrial degeneration and vesiculation of the outer cell membrane of the organ of Corti[37] (Fig. 6–10). Since there is evidence that cholesterol synthesis occurs in the crypt cells, their damage may explain the marked cholesterol-lowering effect of neomycin.[36] Direct toxicity to the mucosal cell probably accounts for the steatorrhea, although an interaction between neomycin and bile salts may be a minor contributory factor by interfering with the intraluminal phase of fat digestion.[55]

Oral and, less often, intravenous clindamycin produces pseudomembranous colitis and a proctitis with the unique proctoscopic finding of elevated, cream-colored plaques measuring 2 to 8 mm in diameter, superimposed on a red, friable, edematous mucosa.[31] These plaques are composed of fibrinoid material, polymorphonuclear leukocytes, and epithelial debris but contain no pathogenic bacteria or fungi.[122] They are usually confined to the rectum and sigmoid, may give a characteristic picture on x-ray (Fig. 6–11), and are accompanied by fever, severe diarrhea, and abdominal cramping pain. The granularity of ulcerative colitis is not seen. A similar picture is produced by lincomycin. The symptoms of colitis may begin and last for weeks after the drug has been stopped.

Metabolic System

The diamidine compounds, of which pentamidine is a member, were originally developed as hypoglycemic agents.[106] Hypoglycemia may be responsible for apparent neurotoxicity during or soon after pentamidine

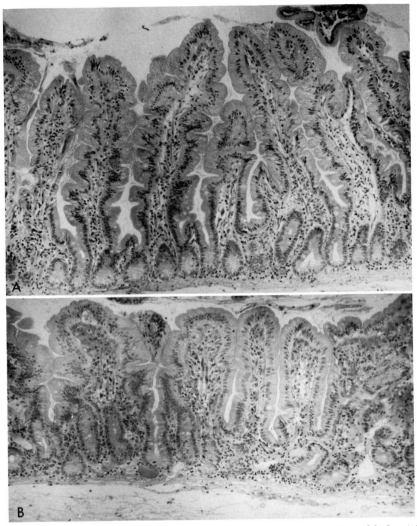

Figure 6–10. Comparison of intestinal biopsies from the same patient obtained before (A) and after (B) eight days of treatment with oral neomycin. After neomycin the villi are shortened and there is infiltration of the lamina propria by round cells and macrophages. (From Dobbins WO, et al: Morphologic alterations associated with neomycin induced malabsorption. Am J Med Sci 255:67, 1968.)

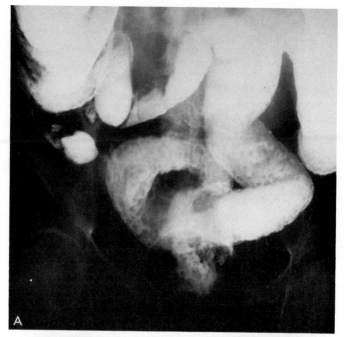

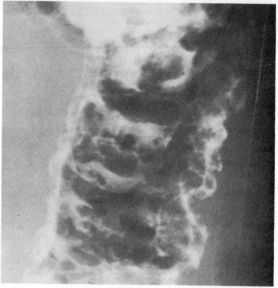

Figure 6–11. A, Barium enema showing plaque-like mucosal lesions throughout sigmoid colon. No ulcerations are seen. These findings are absent in ulcerative colitis and are virtually diagnostic of pseudomembranous colitis. *B,* Air contrast enema also shows the numerous rounded plaques crowding the mucosa in clindamycin-associated pseudomembranous colitis. (From Tedesco FI, et al: Diagnostic features of clindamycin-associated pseudomembranous colitis. N Engl J Med 290:842, 1974.)

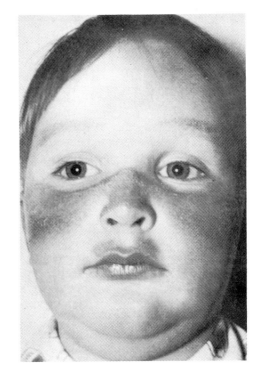

Figure 6–12. Photosensitivity due to chlortetracycline produced malar erythema in this fair-skinned child. (From Verhagen ARHB: Photosensitivity due to chlortetracycline. Dermatologica *130*:440, 1965, published by S. Karger AG, Basel, Switzerland.)

therapy for *Pneumocystis* infection or African sleeping sickness. In doses used for prophylaxis of *Trypanosoma gambiense* infections, no toxicity has been noted.

Skin

Nalidixic acid, griseofulvin, chlortetracycline, and demethylchlortetracycline cause photosensitivity.[110, 123, 132] This reaction is probably phototoxic rather than photoallergic. It can range from intense sunburn and loosening of the nails with the use of the tetracyclines to bullous skin eruptions, with nalidixic acid (Table 6–4). These phototoxic reactions probably result from the conversion of the drug by light to a noxious agent. The reactions begin soon after the start of treatment, occur only at the site of sun exposure, and do not spread to covered areas (Fig. 6–12). The ultraviolet sensitivity to the tetracyclines may persist for weeks after the drugs have been stopped. For unknown reasons, chlorination makes the tetracyclines phototoxic. Demethylchlortetracycline is much more phototoxic than chlortetracycline, producing reactions with ordinary doses in white patients. The phototoxicity of chlortetracycline, on the other hand, becomes evident only with high doses and is more common in young children with fair skin. The greater phototoxicity of demethylchlortetracycline seems related to the absence of a methyl group in the 6-position on the basic tetracycline molecule.

Deposition of Tetracyclines in Teeth and Bones

The tetracyclines localize in growing bone and developing teeth. When given during the last trimester of pregnancy, tetracycline deposits as a fluorescent compound throughout the human fetal skeleton. In premature infants it may cause reversible depression of normal skeletal growth.[32] Deposition of tetracyclines in the teeth of fetuses and in the teeth of infants during the first six to eight years of life can produce permanent discoloration and enamel defects. In general, permanent teeth show less tetracycline effect because the thicker, darker, and more opaque permanent teeth can hide the bands of tetracycline complex laid down in the enamel and dentin.[50] Table 6–4 summarizes the direct toxic effects of antimicrobial drugs on the liver, bowel, skin, and teeth.

Cardiovascular System

Only two antimicrobials have well-established direct toxicity on the heart, and both are antiparasitic. Emetine can cause hypotension and precordial pain. The toxicity to the myocardium is evident from abnormal electrocardiograms where flattened or inverted T waves occur in all leads, and the Q-T interval is prolonged.[100] These disturbances are said to occur in 25 to 50 per cent of patients and require cessation of the drug. Fortunately, metronidazole, which has replaced emetine as the drug of choice for treating amebic liver abscess, is not cardiotoxic. Quinine is the other antimicrobial that is toxic to cardiac muscle. It depresses conduction velocity and contractility, and is especially dangerous in patients with auricular fibrillation or flutter because, like quinidine, it reduces the degree of atrioventricular block and facilitates ventricular tachycardia.

HYPERSENSITIVITY (ALLERGIC) REACTIONS

Mechanisms and Manifestations of Penicillin Allergy

These are the result of an immune reaction between an antigenic derivative of the drug and a specific antibody or sensitized lymphocyte (Table 6–5). Sensitization requires an induction period of five to seven days after the first exposure. The symptoms are those of classical allergy, and they are reproduced upon rechallenge. Nearly every antimicrobial drug can cause allergic reactions by these criteria, but the mechanisms have been extensively studied only with respect to penicillin.

Like other simple chemicals, penicillin and its derivatives are haptens that must combine irreversibly with a carrier molecule in order to become immunogenic and induce hypersensitivity. Conjugation may occur before injection with carriers present as contaminants in penicillin solutions or after injection in vivo by formation of chemical bonds with proteins. The carriers are usually proteins but can be peptides and polysaccharides. This reaction between antibiotic haptens and protein carriers is different from

TABLE 6–5.   *Specificity of Immunologic Reactions to Penicillin*

Type of Reaction	Immunoglobulin	Hapten
Anaphylaxis	IgE	Benzylpenicilloyl
Urticaria		Benzylpenicillin
		Benzylpenicilloate and other minor determinants
Coombs' positive hemolytic anemia	IgG	Benzylpenicilloyl
Serum sickness syndrome and vasculitis	IgG	Benzylpenicilloyl
Interstitial nephritis	IgG	Dimethoxyphenylpenicilloyl Benzylpenicilloyl
Morbilliform eruptions	IgM	Benzylpenicilloyl Minor determinants (?)
Blocking antibodies	IgG	Benzylpenicilloyl Minor determinants

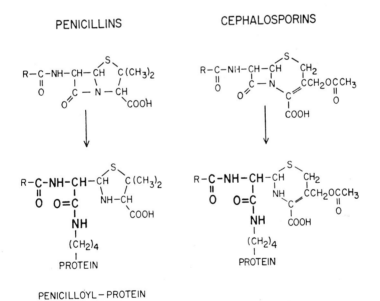

PENICILLINS

CEPHALOSPORINS

PENICILLOYL – PROTEIN
CONJUGATE

Figure 6–13.   Change in chemical structure of penicillins and cephalosporins involved in the formation of reactive compounds capable of conjugating with protein carriers. The protein conjugate is formed here after direct opening of the β-lactam ring of either the penicillin or cephalosporin. Note the identical sections of each conjugate, which are probably the common combining sites for cross-reacting antibodies. (From VanArsdel PP: Serum antibodies to red cell conjugates in penicillin allergy. *In* Penicillin Allergy: Clinical and Immunologic Aspects. Edited by Stewart GT, McGovern JB, 1970, p. 75. Courtesy of Charles C Thomas, Publisher, Springfield, Ill.)

the reversible combination reaction between antibiotics and proteins described in Chapter 5. The hapten-carrier interaction forms a stable covalent bond by electron sharing between the antibiotic residue and an amino acid of the protein. Formation of the covalent bond involves a change in the chemical structure of penicillin to yield reactive compounds capable of conjugating with carriers. The most important penicillin derivative causing penicillin allergy appears to be the penicilloyl determinant, which is designated the *major* determinant of penicillin allergy. One way for penicilloyl-protein conjugates to occur is by direct opening of the β-lactam ring, as shown in Figure 6–13. Another is via penicillenic acid and penicillenic acid derivatives (Fig. 6–14). Penicillenic acid accumulates in aqueous solutions of benzylpenicillin stored at room temperature or in the refrigerator as the pH of the unbuffered solution falls. After injection the penicillenic acid can react with free amino groups and form penicilloyl amide linkages with serum proteins. It is also possible that during the manufacture of penicillin, protein extracted with penicillin from the fermentation medium would form penicilloyl-protein conjugates appearing in the commercial product. This was undoubtedly an important problem before highly purified crystalline benzylpenicillin became available, and has become a serious possibility again in the preparation of 6-aminopenicillanic acid during the manufacture of the newer semisynthetic penicillins. The penicilloylated protein is derived from the *E. coli* preparation employed for the enzymatic removal of the acyl side chain from benzylpenicillin.

While most of the penicillin that undergoes irreversible binding to protein can be identified as benzylpenicilloyl, minor amounts are bound as other haptens and designated *minor determinants*. Two of these minor determinants have been identified as benzylpenicillin itself and sodium benzylpenicilloate, but the chemical nature of the others is unknown. They may participate in penicillin allergy as either immunogens (sensitizers) or elicitors of allergic reactions.[76] Both major and minor determinants can accumulate after storage of penicillin solutions or may be produced *in vivo* after injection.

After a patient has been sensitized to a penicillin-derived hapten, anaphylactic reactions may be elicited by conjugates of low molecular weight. The essential requirement for eliciting an anaphylactic reaction is a minimum of two antigenic determinants per molecule. When two or more penicillin molecules are joined in solution to produce a dimer or polymer, multivalent antigens may be formed without conjugation to a protein carrier. Such dimers or polymers accumulating in penicillin solutions may be responsible for most anaphylactic reactions to penicillin.[34] A stored neutral solution of a good commercial penicillin contains predominantly elicitors of low molecular weight. Anaphylaxis elicited by penicillin derivatives seems to occur through the same mechanism proposed for other antigens. In other words, penicillin anaphylaxis is probably mediated by skin-sensitizing antibodies of the IgE class (reagins) which can attach firmly to the surface of tissue mast cells and basophils. When a divalent or polyvalent penicillin-derived hapten bridges two or more adjacent combin-

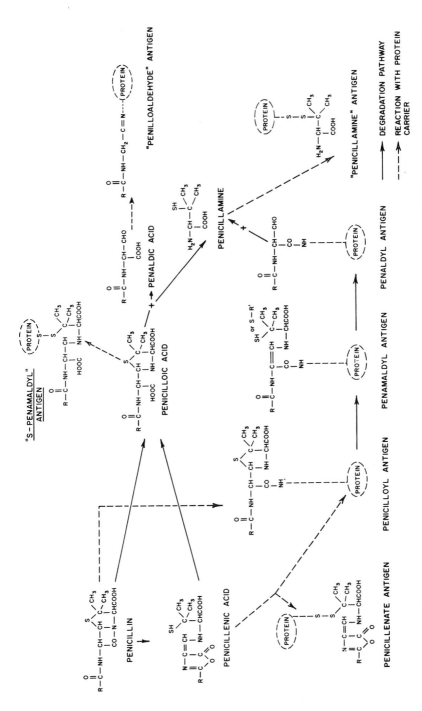

Figure 6–14. Immunochemical pathways leading to the formation of penicillenic acid, penicillenic acid derivatives, and other antigens from penicillin. (From de Weck AL: Drug reactions. *In* Immunological Diseases, 2nd ed. Vol. 1. Edited by Samter M. Boston, Little Brown and Co., 1971, p. 431.)

ing sites of IgE on the surface of these cells, they discharge their intracellular granules and release histamine.

Since human skin-sensitizing antibodies to penicillin have been shown to be specific for the benzylpenicilloyl haptenic determinants and for the minor haptenic determinants, skin-sensitizing antibodies can be detected in patients by skin testing with these antigens. Conjugation of penicillenic acid with lysine polymers gives rise to benzylpenicilloyl-polylysine (BPL), which can be used safely for skin testing in subjects with penicillin allergy and is considerably more sensitive for detecting allergic individuals than is penicillin G.[22] Minor determinant antigens for skin testing can be prepared by dissolving crystalline potassium penicillin G, sodium benzylpenicilloate, and benzylpenicilloic acid, each at 1×10^{-2} M concentration in buffered saline at pH 7.5.[124] Simultaneous skin testing with both major and minor determinant antigens is said to be a promising technique for predicting immediate (2 to 30 minutes) anaphylactic or accelerated (1 to 72 hours) urticarial reactions (with wheezing, pharyngeal edema, or local inflammation) to penicillin.[124] Negative immediate skin tests to these two antigenic preparations virtually exclude the possibility of an anaphylactic reaction and markedly reduce the probability of an accelerated urticarial reaction to penicillin. On the other hand, an immediate wheal and flare reaction to the major and minor determinants after skin pricks or intradermal injection indicates a high probability of immediate or accelerated reaction to penicillins, especially when penicillin is given in high dosages.[78]

Despite the presence of skin-sensitizing antibodies of the IgE class, treatment with penicillin may not cause a reaction. One explanation for this discrepancy is that IgG antibodies, which are present in virtually all patients with positive immediate skin tests to BPL, act as "blocking" antibodies. These IgG blocking antibodies do not mediate anaphylaxis or urticarial reactions themselves but can compete with IgE for antigen. Another explanation is that univalent haptens derived from penicillin can block antibody-combining sites and prevent divalent or multivalent haptens from bridging IgE receptors on mast cells. The monovalent benzylpenicilloyl derivative (N-ϵ-benzylpenicilloyl-N-α-formyl-L-lysine), for example, can inhibit specifically immunologic reactions to penicillin *in vitro* and *in vivo*, including clinical allergic reactions to penicillin in man[35] (Fig. 6–15). The spontaneous development of such monovalent haptens in penicillin preparations might account for the failure of reactions in previously sensitized patients. Deliberate administration of a standardized monovalent hapten might be used as a practical approach to the prevention of penicillin allergy. These blocking antibodies and haptens may explain the low incidence of penicillin-produced anaphylaxis; for, despite the widespread administration of penicillin, not more than 0.04 per cent of patients develop anaphylaxis, while 0.6 per cent have other reactions (especially urticaria). Moreover, only one death has occurred in 94,655 patients treated with penicillin in venereal disease clinics.[108] It should be noted that negative skin tests do not rule out the subsequent occurrence of morbilliform

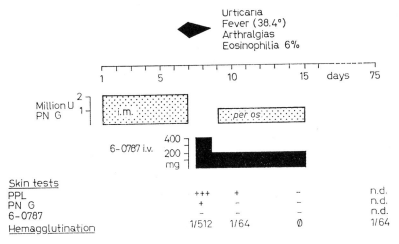

Figure 6–15. Arrest of penicillin reaction (urticaria, fever, arthralgias) by intravenous administration of a monovalent benzylpenicilloyl derivative (designated 6-0787). The duration and severity of the reaction are indicated by the diamond-shaped figure at the top of the diagram. The univalent hapten can block antibody-combining sites and prevent divalent haptens from bridging IgE receptors on mast cells. (From de Weck AL, Girard JP: Specific inhibition of allergic reactions to penicillin in man by a monovalent hapten. Int Arch Allergy 42:801, 1972. Published by S. Karger AG, Basel, Switzerland.)

allergic reactions to penicillin, because these eruptions seem to be mediated by IgM antibodies rather than IgE skin-sensitizing antibodies.[77] Similarly, negative skin tests do not rule out late urticarial reactions that might develop as a result of immune reactions induced during a long course of penicillin therapy.

IgG not only can prevent anaphylaxis and urticarial reactions to penicillin by serving as a blocking antibody, but can also cause harmful immune reactions. IgG mediates hemolytic anemia, the serum sickness syndrome from penicillin, and probably methicillin-associated interstitial nephritis as well. The hemolytic reaction develops when high doses of penicillin are given intravenously before or after intramuscular penicillin. Immunization by both routes of administration seems necessary for coupling benzylpenicilloyl groups to red blood cells and for the formation of high titers of IgG antibodies to benzylpenicilloyl. Benzylpenicilloyl-specific antibodies in the plasma react with the benzylpenicilloyl coupled to red blood cells and produce heavy coating with IgG immunoglobulins,[75] a positive Coombs' test, and the peripheral destruction of red blood cells. The hemolytic anemia disappears after penicillin treatment is stopped, because penicillin-induced antibodies will no longer attach to red blood cells if penicilloylated cells have disappeared from the circulation. These mechanisms also induce hemolytic reactions during cephalothin therapy.[47]

A similar reaction between methicillin antigens and kidney proteins seems to cause interstitial nephritis in patients given large doses of intravenous methicillin. The secretion of methicillin by the proximal renal tubules exposes the structural proteins of the tubular basement membrane to concentrations of the antibiotic high enough to promote hapten-protein conjugates. Antibodies to these conjugates have been shown to react with the carrier portion of the conjugate.[15] Antitubular basement membrane antibodies were detected by indirect immunofluorescence in the serum of a patient who sustained severe renal failure while he was receiving methicillin. IgG, C3, and a methicillin antigen assumed to be dimethoxyphenylpenicilloyl were present in a linear pattern along the tubular basement, but not along the glomerular basement membrane (Fig. 6–16). Antibody to tubular basement membrane has not been detectable when sought in the sera of patients without nephritis during treatment with methicillin, and methicillin antigen did not bind to tubular basement membrane in biopsies of their kidneys. These limited observations suggest that only selected individual patients can develop dimethoxyphenylpenicilloyl conjugates with tubular basement membrane proteins and the immune responses with antitubular basement membrane antibodies that are essential for interstitial nephritis.

The clinical syndrome of methicillin nephritis fits with an allergic mechanism because the fever, rash, eosinophilia, proteinuria, azotemia, and acidosis develop only after high doses (20 to 24 gm daily) are given for at least eight days (Fig. 6–17). The interstitial infiltrate contains large numbers of mononuclear cells and eosinophils and is accompanied by

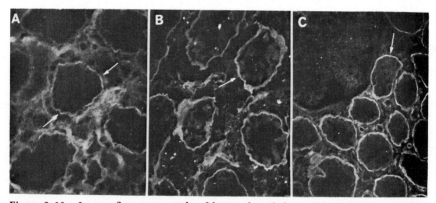

Figure 6–16. Immunofluorescent study of biopsy from kidney with methicillin nephritis. IgG, accompanied by C3, is present circumferentially in a linear pattern (arrows) around most cortical tubules in A. A methicillin antigen (B) assumed to be dimethoxyphenylpenicilloyl is also present along the tubular basement membranes (arrow) of most cortical tubules in the biopsy. IgG, reactive with tubular basement membranes but not glomerular basement membrane, is present in the patient's serum on testing by direct immunofluorescence on normal human kidney in C. These findings suggest that methicillin nephritis occurs in certain patients who first develop dimethoxyphenylpenicilloyl conjugates with the proteins of tubular basement membranes, and then produce antibodies against their own tubular basement membranes. (From Border WA, et al: Antitubular basement-membrane antibodies in methicillin-associated interstitial nephritis. N Engl J Med 291:383, 1974.)

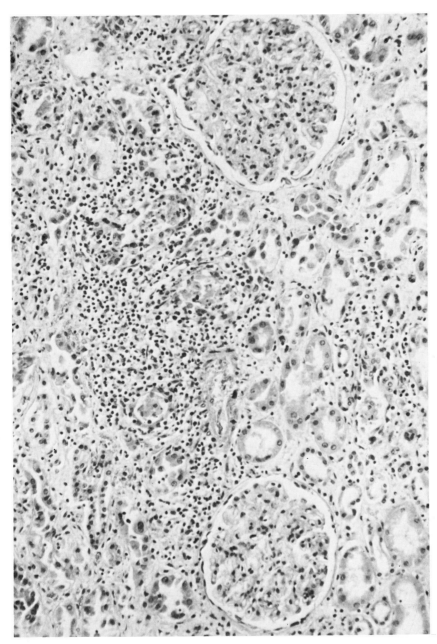

Figure 6–17. Clinical course of methicillin nephropathy. Fever, eosinophilia, and azotemia subsided soon after methicillin was stopped. Renal biopsy showed irregular interstitial accumulation of leukocytes and tubular damage. The infiltrate contained large numbers of mononuclear cells and eosinophils. (From Baldwin DS, et al: Renal failure and interstitial nephritis due to penicillin and methicillin. N Engl J Med 279:1248, 1968.)

tubular damage without glomerular abnormalities or arteritis. The same syndrome of interstitial nephritis has been described after continuous high doses of benzylpenicillin (20 million units daily), other penicillins, cephalosporins, and sulfonamides[8, 24, 25] (Fig. 6–18). In most patients the process is reversible, but death has occurred from renal failure.

The serum sickness syndrome usually begins 5 to 14 days after the start of penicillin therapy with generalized urticaria, fever, joint swelling, and lymphadenopathy. Urticaria is probably mediated by IgE skin-sensitizing antibodies and the other manifestations by immune complexes formed between penicillin derivatives and IgG. More rarely, these complexes may be the basis, after penicillin therapy, for vasculitis of the skin, kidney, gastrointestinal tract, lung, and nervous system.

Although most observations on allergy to the penicillins have been made with benzylpenicillin, the information obtained applies to many semisynthetic penicillins. For example, immunologic cross reactions occur between haptens prepared from various semisynthetic penicillins. The extent of cross reactivity varies not only with the semisynthetic penicillin but also with individual sera. Extensive cross reactions have been noted between the penicilloyl haptens of benzylpenicillin and ampicillin, but only

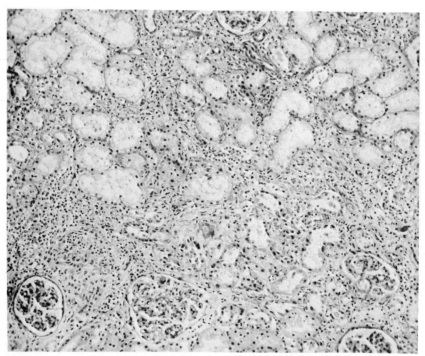

Figure 6–18. Interstitial nephritis attributed to cephalothin therapy. These findings were present 60 days after cephalothin was discontinued. There is interstitial mononuclear infiltration, mild edema, and early fibrosis with patchy tubular atrophy. The glomeruli and proximal tubules are spared. (From Burton JR, et al: Acute renal failure during cephalothin therapy. JAMA 229:681, 1974.)

slight cross reactions occur between the haptens of benzylpenicillin and those of methicillin or oxacillin.[72] In other words, the side group of the penicillin molecule affects its immunologic behavior. The importance of side groups is also noted in studies on the primary immunogenicity of penicillin preparations. Phenethicillin, for example, an acid-stable phenoxy derivative (syncillin), is far less immunogenic than benzylpenicillin and methicillin, apparently because penicillins with the phenoxy side group do not form significant amounts of penicillenic acids.[40]

Penicillins also cross react with cephalosporins experimentally, but the significance of such reactions in patients has not been settled. When the cephalosporin antibiotics were introduced, it was hoped that their structural differences from the penicillins would avoid such cross reactions (compare Figs. 1–1, 1–2, 1–3, and 1–4). The six-membered dihydrothiazine ring of cephalosporins differs from the five-membered thiazolidine ring of penicillin, and the side chain structures of most cephalosporins differ from those of the penicillins. (Ampicillin is an exception because its side chain is similar to that of cephalexin.) Most clinical evidence indicates that this hope has materialized and that, although a few reports of anaphylaxis on first exposure to cephalosporins have appeared,[111] cephalosporins can be safely taken by patients sensitive to penicillin.[120] Cephalosporins and penicillins have cross-reacting major antigenic determinants, the cephalosporyl and penicilloyl groups, but their minor antigenic determinants do not cross react readily.[5] In view of the limited cross reactivity between the haptens, the great variability among individual antisera in extent of cross reactivity, and the proved safety of cephalosporins in many patients who have experienced severe allergic reactions to penicillin, it would appear that cephalosporins should not be withheld when treatment of the infection warrants their use in patients who exhibit serious hypersensitivity to penicillin.

Management of Penicillin Allergy

If cephalosporins cannot be substituted in patients with life-threatening infections, desensitization to penicillin can be considered for severe penicillin allergy based on history and skin tests. The results of skin testing with major and minor determinants will indicate how the desensitization should be done. Those reacting only to the major determinant, benzylpenicilloyl-polylysine, can be desensitized rapidly, while reactions to minor determinants warrant slow desensitization. The rapid "desensitization" probably depends on blocking antibodies, while slow desensitization to minor determinant hypersensitivity is probably true desensitization because there is a complete disappearance of reagin and patients can tolerate high-dosage penicillin therapy for weeks.[73]

Before hypersensitization or desensitization is started, equipment and drugs for treating anaphylaxis should be brought to the bedside. The most important of these drugs is epinephrine (aqueous, 1:1000) given in a dose of

0.5 ml intramuscularly. Aminophylline and hydrocortisone may be of some value after the administration of epinephrine. Equipment for an emergency tracheotomy and for oxygen administration is also necessary.

Intravenous fluid should be started and, with a physician in attendance, penicillin should be administered subcutaneously in the distal portion of the extremity so that a tourniquet can be applied if necessary. The beginning dose of penicillin is 5 units, and it is doubled every 15 minutes. After a dose of 100,000 units, the intravenous route is used for initiation of therapeutic doses of penicillin. Until then, the blood, pulse, and respiration should be determined at five-minute intervals.[48]

Antihistamines are of no proved value in preventing or treating anaphylactic reactions but do help control urticaria and other allergic reactions to penicillin. The same is true for corticosteroids. They are of dubious value for penicillin anaphylaxis but can suppress many other effects of penicillin allergy, especially the serum sickness type of reaction.

If morbilliform or urticarial eruptions occur during therapy with penicillin, the drug can be continued because the risk of a serious allergic reaction is small. In the majority of patients the urticaria will disappear despite continued administration of penicillin, because either IgG blocking antibodies develop or reagin production stops.[74] Morbilliform reactions to penicillin also disappear in most patients while the drug is still being administered. Ampicillin produces the highest incidence of morbilliform eruptions, 3 to 8 per cent, and this reaches 50 to 80 per cent in patients with infectious mononucleosis. These ampicillin rashes are probably not immunologic in origin. Erythema nodosum, erythema multiforme, purpura, and vesiculobullous reactions are seen only rarely in association with penicillin therapy.

Hypersensitivity to Antimicrobial Drugs Other Than Penicillin

All the immunologic reactions described for penicillin can occur with other antimicrobial drugs. The aminoglycosides, tetracycline, and chloramphenicol have all been associated with anaphylactic reactions. The serum sickness syndrome was common when sulfadiazine and sulfathiazole were used in large doses to treat meningitis. Drug fever can be a consequence of treatment with nearly any antimicrobial. One mechanism for drug fever is circulating immune complexes, as in the serum sickness pattern of drug reaction. It is also possible that drug fever might be a manifestation of delayed hypersensitivity and might be mediated through a substance released upon contact between drug and sensitized lymphocyte.[6]

Besides causing hemolytic anemia, immunologic processes are involved in the production of thrombocytopenic purpura and agranulocytosis by antimicrobial drugs. The lactam antibiotics, streptomycin, the sulfonamides, chloroquine, isoniazid, stibophen, and rifampin have been implicated in immunologic platelet destruction, but only quinine, stibophen, and rifampin have convincingly been shown to operate through an immunologic mechanism involving a reaction between the drug and its antibody.[102] The best available evidence indicates that the drug binds to a carrier to form the primary antigen, which stimulates drug-specific antibody. The drug-antibody complex then coats platelets so that they are destroyed as "innocent bystanders."[115] It is theoretically possible that such complexes may attach to other cells, thus providing a general explanation for immunologic injury by antimicrobial drugs. This mechanism has not been clearly established for neutrophil injury, and relatively little is known about the immunologic basis of agranulocytosis secondary to antimicrobials. The penicillins, streptomycin, and the sulfonamides have been associated with agranulocytic reactions that were thought to have an immunologic basis, but the nature of the injury to neutrophils is obscure.

While skin eruptions, anaphylaxis, and blood disorders are the main allergic reactions to antimicrobials, the liver and lung may also occasionally be involved. Isoniazid hepatitis, discussed earlier in this chapter, is thought to be caused by hypersensitivity. The same is true of the cholestatic jaundice secondary to erythromycin estolate. Premonitory symptoms of abdominal cramps, nausea, and vomiting are followed by fever, leukocytosis, and eosinophilia. Symptoms and findings subside within three to five days after the erythromycin estolate has been stopped, with reinstitution of the antibiotic producing a return of the syndrome.[18] The hepatotoxic property seems to reside in the propionyl ester linkage at the 2'-position, and cross sensitivity has not been observed with plain erythromycin, erythromycin stearate, erythromycin gluceptate, or erythromycin ethyl succinate[122] (Fig. 6–19).

Nitrofurantoin causes the most distinctive type of pulmonary disease attributed to hypersensitivity among antimicrobials.[53] Approximately 200 cases of pulmonary sensitivity reactions to nitrofurantoin have been reported since 1959 (Fig. 6–20). These reactions produce a nonfatal syndrome of acute febrile, noncardiac, pulmonary edema with cough, dysp-

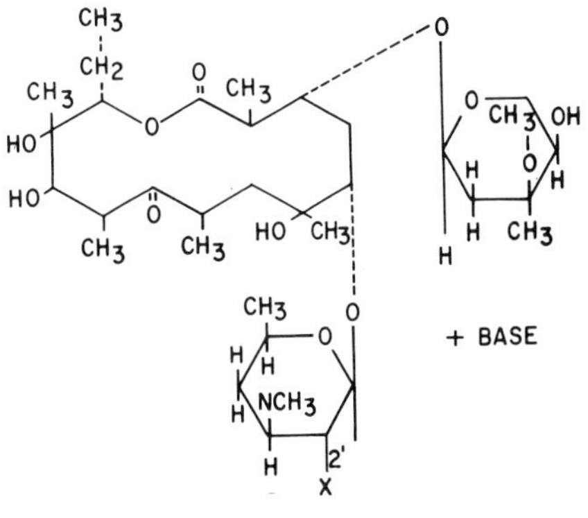

Figure 6-19. Chemical structure of erythromycin. The ester linkage of propionic acid at the 2'-position seems to be responsible for the hepatotoxicity of erythromycin compounds. (From Tolman KG, et al: Chemical structure of erythromycin and hepatotoxicity. Ann Intern Med 81:59, 1974.)

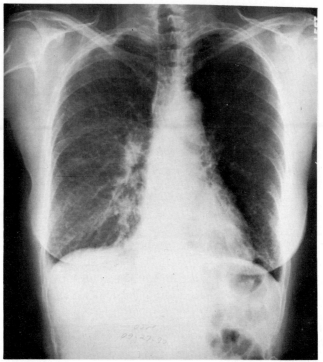

Figure 6–20. Acute nitrofurantoin pneumonitis in a 54-year-old woman patient who received nitrofurantoin for one week and developed an eruption over the entire body. The x-ray findings are those of interstitial edema in the presence of normal heart size and normal vascularity of the upper lobe. There are marked Kerley lines, especially Kerley B lines, in the periphery of the right lung.

nea, eosinophilia, and, sometimes, pleural effusions. Patients recover rapidly when the drug is withdrawn. About 3 per cent experience subacute or chronic reactions that develop into diffuse interstitial pneumonitis or fibrosis after prolonged treatment with nitrofurantoin. In contrast to the acute nitrofurantoin lung reaction, the chronic process begins insidiously without fever. The chronic form is at least partly reversible if the drug is stopped before extensive interstitial fibrosis has developed. Steroids may be necessary to reverse the interstitial pneumonitis.[107]

In contrast to drugs that cause trouble through allergic mechanisms, at least one antibiotic, rifampin, appears to inhibit hypersensitivity reactions.[51] Rifampin can reduce or abolish the tuberculin reactions in patients and suppress the activity of T lymphocytes (Fig. 6–21). T-lymphocyte suppression occurs within two to three weeks after institution of rifampin therapy and is completely reversible after withdrawal of the drug. The immunosuppressive effect does not seem to hinder the effectiveness of the drug in the treatment of patients with tuberculosis.

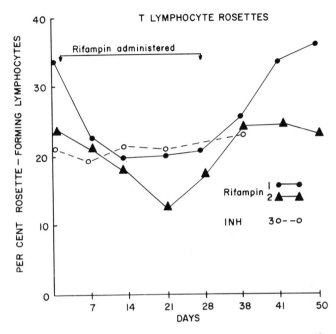

Figure 6–21. Suppression of T lymphocytes by rifampin. Rifampin suppresses T-lymphocyte rosette formation. Serial T-lymphocyte rosettes were studied in two subjects (1 and 2) receiving rifampin, 600 mg daily, for 28 days and in one subject (3) receiving isoniazid (INH), 300 mg daily, for 38 days. (From Gupta S, Grieco MH, Siegel I: Suppression of T-lymphocyte rosettes of rifampin. Ann Intern Med 82:486, 1975.)

TOXIC REACTIONS ATTRIBUTED
TO MICROBIAL LYSIS

Effective drug therapy of infection sometimes causes paradoxical worsening of symptoms, presumably because microbial lysis releases toxic products (Table 6–6). These reactions can be serious, but seldom are fatal. One of the most severe is the Jarisch-Herxheimer reaction in syphilis of the brain. Sudden death may occur after penicillin treatment for gumma of the brain is started, and extreme cerebral irritability may complicate the early stages of penicillin therapy for general paresis. The histologic changes encountered in syphilitic lesions during the Jarisch-Herxheimer reaction involve the small blood vessels in an inflammatory process resembling in all respects the tuberculin reaction. This suggests that the reaction from treating syphilis is one of delayed hypersensitivity to antigens released from killed treponemes.[114] Similar reactions occur in the skin and other tissues of patients treated for syphilis and for such spirochetal infections as rat-bite fever (*Spirillum minus*) and relapsing fever (*Borrelia recurrentis*). The reaction occurs with the first dose only and is not a contraindication to further treatment. It can be minimized by withholding treatment during the febrile paroxysm in relapsing fever.

TABLE 6–6. *Adverse Reactions Attributed to Microbial Lysis*

DRUG	INFECTION	TOXIC SIGNS
Penicillin	Syphilis	Jarisch-Herxheimer reaction
Tetracycline	Brucellosis	Increased fever, hypotension
Dapsone	Lepromatous leprosy	Erythema nodosum leprosum
Dapsone	Dimorphous leprosy	Reversal reaction
Diethylcarbamazine	Bancroftian filariasis	Fever, lymphadenopathy, and acute lymphedema
Diethylcarbamazine	Loiasis	Calabar swellings
Diethylcarbamazine	Onchocerciasis	Local pruritus, edema, and ocular inflammation

Among nonspirochetal infections, brucellosis is most likely to produce a systemic type of "Herxheimer" reaction after the start of treatment.[119] The most severe Herxheimer-like reaction occurs in *Brucella melitensis* infections, which show an abrupt rise in fever 12 to 24 hours after treatment is started with a tetracycline. Some of these patients also develop septic shock with hypotension and tachycardia, but the reaction is quickly reversible, and no fatalities have been reported.

Treatment also accentuates the adverse response to leprosy. Up to 50 per cent of patients with lepromatous leprosy given sulfones suffer from erythema nodosum leprosum. Disseminated, tender, inflamed nodules erupt in crops all over the skin. These nodules are accompanied by fever, polyneuritis, glomerulonephritis, iritis, and severe joint pains. Since the nodules have the appearance histologically of the Arthus reaction and occur mainly after three to six months of treatment when massive bacillary death seems to occur, the lesions might be an expression of immune complex vasculitis. Immunoglobulin G and complement (C3) have been demonstrated within these nodular lesions.[126] The "reversal" reaction is seen during treatment of dimorphous leprosy but is less common than erythema nodosum. In dimorphous (or borderline) leprosy some of the lesions resemble the lepromatous form of leprosy and others resemble the tuberculoid form. The "reversal" reaction of borderline leprosy seems to represent a restoration of cellular immunity manifested by an increased number of lymphocytes in the lesions and a decline in the number of bacilli. Existing lesions become acutely inflamed and may develop bullae or ulcers. Severe nerve damage occurs as the neuritis rapidly advances. Both erythema nodosum and reversal reactions can be controlled by corticosteroids in severe cases, while chloroquine and aspirin are effective in milder reactions. Thalidomide can completely suppress erythema nodosum leprosum, but because it is teratogenic, its use is limited to men and to women beyond the childbearing age.

Among nonbacterial infections, therapeutic reactions to microbial killing are seen mainly in filariasis. The death of microfilaria or adult worms during treatment of bancroftian filariasis, onchocerciasis, and loiasis with diethylcarbamazine (Hetrazan) may lead to severe allergic reactions. In bancroftian filariasis, the destruction of microfilaria and adult worms may cause headache, fever, and the painful swelling of lymph nodes. Swollen nodules containing dead adult worms appear along the lymphatics and are sometimes the site of lymphatic blockade, with transient hydrocoele and lymphedema. Most patients with loaisis develop allergic reactions in the subcutaneous lesions (calabar swellings), as microfilaria and adult worms are destroyed during the first few days of treatment. In addition to headache and arthralgias, local pruritus, edema, and, occasionally, new calabar swellings appear. In onchocerciasis the adult worm is not killed, but allergic reactions to the killing of microfilaria by diethylcarbamazine develop. These symptoms reach their height in 12 to 15 hours and may be so bad that the treatment seems worse than the disease. Patients experience not only fever, joint pains, and inflamed pruritic skin, but are also in danger of losing their sight because of ocular inflammation. Starting treatment with small doses of diethylcarbamazine and antihistamines helps to minimize the reactions. Steroids are useful in treatment of these reactions to killed filaria in all three forms of filariasis.

CHANGE IN MICROBIAL FLORA

Most antibiotics change the character of the indigenous microflora on the mucous membranes and skin. This was first observed when oral penicillin caused a replacement of gram-positive bacteria with coliform bacilli; when the drug was stopped, the normal flora returned. The extent of the change and its pathologic potential vary with the antimicrobial drug, its dosage, and the underlying resistance of the patient. Claims have been made that superinfections resulting from antibiotic therapy are a serious cause of pneumonia due to gram-negative bacilli.[54] Critical examination of this problem has opened to question the importance of antibiotics in causing superinfections, because the colonization of the oropharynx by gram-negative bacilli increases markedly in severely ill patients who are not receiving antibiotics.[61] Since most bacterial pneumonias begin with aspiration of bacteria from the upper respiratory tract, this change in pharyngeal flora brought on by sickness alone could account for pneumonia due to gram-negative bacilli in hospitalized patients (Fig. 6–22).

There are, however, at least two unequivocal infectious complications related to eliminating normal flora with antibiotics. One of these is mucocutaneous candidiasis, which can be brought on by any antibiotic but especially by tetracycline, ampicillin, and certain combinations that inhibit a wide spectrum of normally resident bacteria. The mere increase in the number of *Candida* on body surfaces that often occurs after antibiotic treatment does not in itself have any clinical significance and does not warrant a diagnosis of candidiasis. The commonest forms of candidiasis after the use of antibiotics are vaginitis and oral thrush.[45,118]

Prolongation of *Salmonella* carriage is the other well-documented complication of eliminating competitive microflora.[4] Antibiotic therapy in

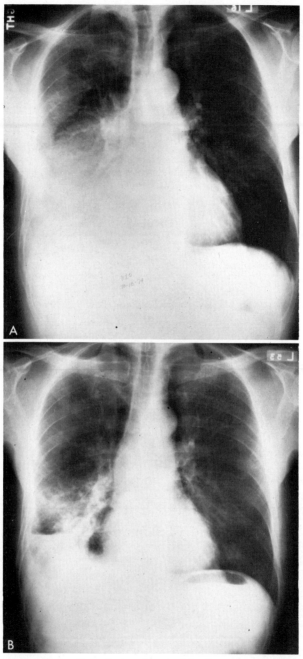

Figure 6–22. Superinfection lung abscess due to *Klebsiella pneumoniae* in patient treated with 800,000 units penicillin G daily for pneumococcal pneumonia. *A,* Chest x-ray showing pneumonia before lung abscess. *B,* Chest x-ray showing *Klebsiella* lung abscess.

acute *Salmonella* gastroenteritis prolongs postconvalescent excretion and increases the opportunity for spread from one person to another. This problem develops despite continued susceptibility of the *Salmonella* to the antibiotics and is best explained by preferential suppression of the more susceptible bacteria of the normal gut and their replacement by salmonellae.

DRUG INTERACTIONS

Adverse interactions between drugs may occur when they are mixed in intravenous solutions during administration, or after their administration by the same or different routes. The number of drug incompatibilities in solution is too large to list here, but some important ones are given in Table 6–7. This table also lists most of the drug interactions that can occur in the patient after administration.

Drug incompatibilities in solution take the form of inactivation or precipitation. Methicillin quickly loses its activity after mixing with kanamycin, and gentamicin is slowly inactivated by carbenicillin. Half the activity of gentamicin is lost after 8 to 12 hours of incubation with carbenicillin in physiologic saline.[90,104] Ampicillin produces a 50 per cent loss of gentamicin activity in two hours, but the other penicillins and cephalosporins do not cause significant inactivation of gentamicin[97] (Fig. 6–23). Examples of inactivation or precipitation by solutes in solution are given in Table 6–7. The importance of pH is illustrated by benzylpenicillin, which is stable for 12 hours at pH 5.5 to 6.5 but unstable in dextrose solution at alkaline pH. Its activity is rapidly lost at a pH below 5.5 or 7.5. Methicillin and nafcillin are also inactivated at acid pH and require buffering. Tetracycline, in contrast, requires a very acid pH of 1.8 to 2.8 for maximum stability. Ascorbic acid is used as the stabilizer. Amino acid solutions are unsatisfactory vehicles for antibiotics, but lactated Ringer's solution can be relied on as safe for administering most antibiotics.

In general, erythromycin lactobionate, vancomycin hydrochloride, polymyxin B sulfate, tetracycline hydrochloride, and the lincomycins should not be given in the same solution as another antibiotic because of physical incompatibilities. Two other drugs, heparin and hydrocortisone, also produce incompatible reactions in solution with several antibiotics.

TABLE 6–7.   *Major Drug Interactions in Solution*

DRUGS	EFFECT
Kanamycin and methicillin	Inactivation of methicillin
Gentamicin and ampicillin or carbenicillin	Inactivation of gentamicin
Amphotericin and 0.9% NaCl	Precipitation of amphotericin B
Erythromycin lactobionate and 0.9% NaCl	Precipitation of erythromycin
Penicillins and bicarbonate in 5% dextrose	Inactivation of various penicillins

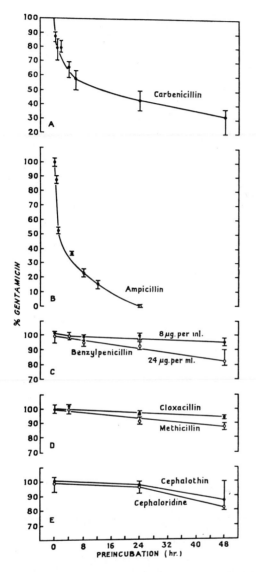

Figure 6–23. Inactivation of gentamicin by carbenicillin and ampicillin. Gentamicin mixed with carbenicillin, ampicillin, benzylpenicillin, methicillin, cloxacillin, cephalothin, or cephaloridine was incubated in intravenous infusion fluids at room temperature. Remaining gentamicin activity is expressed as a percentage of the same concentration of gentamicin incubated alone for the same period in identical solutions. (From Noone P, Pattison JR: Therapeutic implications of interaction of gentamicin and penicillins. Lancet 2:575, 1971.)

Reactions *in vivo* from interactions between drugs administered separately may result from a number of different mechanisms. Rashes from ampicillin increase from 7.5 to 22.4 per cent in patients taking allopurinol, probably because allopurinol potentiates drug allergy, but also possibly because hyperuricemia does so.[60] Interference with anticoagulant therapy occurs in patients given either coumarin derivatives or heparin during therapy with certain antimicrobials. Rifampin and griseofulvin reduce the anticoagulant effect of coumarin drugs, while nalidixic acid, quinine, chloramphenicol, and other broad-spectrum antibiotics cause excessive anticoagulation by the different mechanisms indicated in Table 6–8.[10] These vary from stimulating metabolic degradation (griseofulvin) and reducing

TABLE 6–8. *Major Drug Interactions in Patients*

NATURE OR SITE OF DISTURBANCE	DRUGS	EFFECT
Skin	Ampicillin and allopurinol	Potentiation of ampicillin rashes
Blood cells	Trimethoprim and thiazides or furosemide	Increased incidence of thrombocytopenia
	Trimethoprim/sulfamethoxazole and immunosuppressive drugs	Leukopenia
Clotting	Tetracyclines and heparin	Diminished anticoagulant effect
	Rifampin and coumarin derivatives (Fig. 6–24)	Diminished anticoagulant effect
	Griseofulvin and dicumarol	Stimulates metabolic degradation of dicumarol
	Nalidixic acid and dicumarol	Displaces dicumarol from protein and prolongs prothrombin time
	Quinine and dicumarol	Quinine depresses prothrombin formation and increases anticoagulant effect
	Broad-spectrum antibiotics and dicumarol	Increases anticoagulant effect by depressing vitamin K synthesis in gut
	Chloramphenicol and diphenylhydantoin	Increased toxicity from diphenylhydantoin
	Chloramphenicol and dicumarol	Excessive anticoagulation
Metabolic	Chloramphenicol and tolbutamide	Hypoglycemia
	Sulfaphenizole and tolbutamide	Hypoglycemic attacks
Renal	Cephaloridine and furosemide	Enhanced nephrotoxicity of cephaloridine
	Cephalothin and colistin	Enhanced nephrotoxicity of colistin
	Cephalothin and gentamicin	Enhanced nephrotoxicity of gentamicin
Absorption	Tetracyclines and antacids	Reduced absorption of tetracyclines
	Tetracyclines and iron salts	Reduced absorption of iron salts
Degradation	Doxycycline and barbiturates	Accelerated breakdown of doxycycline·
	Doxycycline and diphenylhydantoin	Accelerated breakdown of doxycycline

protein binding (nalidixic acid) of dicumarol to depressing prothrombin formation directly (quinine) or indirectly by preventing vitamin K synthesis in the intestinal microflora (broad-spectrum antibiotics). Since chloramphenicol interferes with the hepatic transformation of dicumarol, tolbutamide, and diphenylhydantoin, these three drugs can reach toxic levels

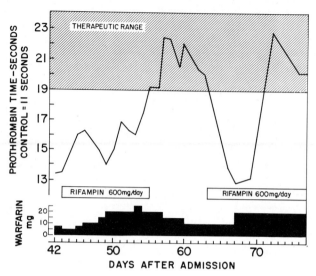

Figure 6–24. Increased warfarin requirement during rifampin therapy. (From Romankiewicz JA, Ehrman M: Rifampin and warfarin: a drug interaction. Ann Intern Med 82:225, 1975.)

in patients under treatment with chloramphenicol.[30] The sulfonamide, sulfaphenizole, is reported to exercise a similar effect in potentiating the activity of tolbutamide so that hypoglycemic attacks occur.[29]

Interference with anticoagulant drug therapy may also result from antagonism of heparin activity by tetracycline. Antacids and iron salts interfere with the absorption of most tetracyclines, while barbiturates and diphenylhydantoin stimulate the metabolic degradation of doxycycline in the liver.[95, 99]

Diuretics enhance the toxicity of at least two antimicrobials. Furosemide potentiates the nephrotoxicity of cephaloridine, while an increased incidence of thrombocytopenia from trimethoprim-sulfamethoxazole has been observed mainly in older patients receiving thiazides or furosemide.[68] Leukopenia from trimethoprim-sulfamethoxazole is more common in patients receiving immunosuppressive drugs.[58]

REACTIONS TO THE PROCAINE AND CATION MOIETY OF PENICILLIN

Not all reactions are attributed to the active moiety of antibiotics. Certain reactions to procaine penicillin, for example, have been blamed on the procaine. These acute reactions occur immediately after intramuscular procaine penicillin and subside in a few minutes. They usually produce neurologic symptoms ranging from dizziness, tinnitus, and headache to grand mal convulsions. Patients also experience fear of imminent death, unusual smells, and visual disturbances. Although these were once thought to be caused by microembolization of the lung and brain, careful studies suggest that they are more likely the result of instantaneous liberation *in vivo* of toxic quantities of procaine.[49] In patients given 4.8 million units of procaine penicillin for the treatment of gonorrhea, plasma procaine concentrations ranged from 3.8 to 11.0 μg/ml.

Cation intoxication may be a serious problem with penicillin and carbenicillin because they are given in high doses intravenously. Most commercially available penicillin G preparations contain 1.5 milliequivalents (mEq) of potassium ion in one million units, and carbenicillin has 4.7 mEq of sodium per gram. The concentration of potassium in penicillin may not produce problems, even though glomerular filtration is greatly reduced, because of the great capacity of distal tubules to secrete potassium into the urine. In oliguric patients, however, serum potassium reaches dangerous levels, and the practice of giving "massive" doses of penicillin might precipitate hyperkalemia. The reverse can occur with large doses of carbenicillin and sodium penicillin. Hypokalemia and metabolic alkalosis may result from large doses of carbenicillin in renal disease because tubular secretion of potassium is enhanced by a high sodium intake.[56] High doses of carbenicillin also provide cardiac patients with excessive sodium. Daily intravenous doses of 20 to 30 gm impose a load of 2 to 3 gm of sodium and could interfere with control of heart failure.

REFERENCES

1. Acocella G, Bonollo L, Garimoldi M, et al: Kinetics of rifampicin and isoniazid administered alone and in combination to normal subjects and patients with liver disease. Gut 13:47–53, 1972.
2. Altman R, Black K, Goldfield M: Vestibular reactions to minocycline after meningococcal prophylaxis. Morbidity and Mortality Weekly Report, US Dept HEW 24:9–11, 1975.
3. Arcieri GM, Falco FG, Smith HM, et al: Clinical research experience with gentamicin. Incidence of adverse reactions. Med J Aust 1:Suppl:30–34, 1970.
4. Aserkoff B, Bennett JV:Effect of antibiotic therapy in acute salmonellosis on the fecal excretion of salmonellae. N Engl J Med 281:636–640, 1969.
5. Assem ES, Vickers MR: Tests for penicillin allergy in man. II. The immunological cross-reaction between penicillins and cephalosporins. Immunology 27:255–269, 1974.
6. Atkins E, Feldman JD, Francis L, et al: Studies on the mechanism of fever accompanying delayed hypersensitivity. The role of the sensitized lymphocyte. J Exp Med 135:1113–1132, 1972.
7. Ayala GF, Lin S, Vasconetto C: Penicillin as epileptogenic agent: Its effect on an isolated neuron. Science 167:1257–1259, 1970.
8. Baldwin DS, Levine BB, McCluskey RT, et al: Renal failure and interstitial nephritis due to penicillin and methicillin. N Engl J Med 279:1245–1252, 1968.
9. Benner EJ: Cephaloridine and the kidneys (editorials). J Infect Dis 122:104–105, 1970.
10. Beran G: Der Einfluss der Rifampizintherapie auf die orale Antikoagulation mit Acenocumarol. Prax Pneumol 26:350–353, 1972 (in German).
11. Beutler, E: Glucose 6-phosphate dehydrogenase deficiency. *In* Hematology. Edited by Williams WJ, Beutler E, Erslev AJ, Rundles RW. New York, McGraw-Hill, 1972, pp. 391–399.
12. Block ER, Bennett JE: Pharmacological studies with 5-fluorocytosine. Antimicrob Agents Chemother 1:476–482, 1972.

13. Bloomer HA, Barton LJ, Maddock RK Jr: Penicillin-induced encephalopathy in uremic patients. JAMA 200:121–123, 1967.
14. Bobrow SN, Jaffe E, Young RC: Anuria and acute tubular necrosis associated with gentamicin and cephalothin. JAMA 222:1546–1547, 1972.
15. Border WA, Lehman DH, Egan JD, et al: Antitubular basement-membrane antibodies in methicillin-associated interstitial nephritis. N Engl J Med 291:381–384, 1974.
16. Brandriss MU, Wolff SM, Moores R, et al: Anemia induced by amphotericin B. JAMA 189:663–666, 1964.
17. Braude AI, Davey P, Siemienski J: Prevention of blood coagulation by antibiotics in vitro. Proc Soc Exp Biol Med 83:160, 1953.
18. Braun P: Hepatotoxicity of erythromycin. J Infect Dis 119:300–306, 1969.
19. Brown CH, Natelson EA, Bradshaw W, et al: The hemostatic defect produced by carbenicillin. N Engl J Med 291:265–270, 1974.
20. Brownlee G, Bushby SR: Chemotherapy and pharmacology of aerosporin, selective gram-negative antibiotic. Lancet 1:127–132, 1948.
21. Brummer DL, et al: Summary of the report of the Ad Hoc Advisory Committee on isoniazid and liver disease. Morbidity and Mortality Weekly Report, US Dept HEW 20:231–234, 1971.
22. Budd MA, Parker CW, Norden CW: Evaluation of intradermal skin tests in penicillin hypersensitivity. JAMA 190:203–205, 1964.
23. Burgess JL, Birchall R: Nephrotoxicity of amphotericin B, with emphasis on changes in tubular function. Am J Med 53:77–84, 1972.
24. Burton JR, Lichtenstein NS, Colvin RB, et al: Acute interstitial nephritis from oxacillin. Johns Hopkins Med J 134:58–61, 1974.
25. Burton JR, Lichtenstein NS, Colvin RB, et al: Acute renal failure during cephalothin therapy. JAMA 229:679–682, 1974.
26. Butler WT, Bennett JE, Alling DW, et al: Nephrotoxicity of amphotericin B, early and late effects in 81 patients. Ann Intern Med 61:175–187, 1964.
27. Butler WT, Cotlove E: Increased permeability of human erythrocytes induced by amphotericin B. J Infect Dis 123:341–350, 1971.
28. Cahal DA: Reactions to nalidixic acid. Br Med J 5461:590, 1965.
29. Christensen LK, Hansen J, Kristensen M: Sulfaphenazole-induced hypoglycaemic attacks in tolbutamide-treated diabetics. Lancet 2:1298–1301, 1963.
30. Christensen LK, Skovsted L: Inhibition of drug metabolism by chloramphenicol. Lancet 2:1397–1399, 1969.
31. Cohen LE, McNeill CJ, Wells RF: Clindamycin-associated colitis. JAMA 223:1379–1380, 1973.
32. Cohlan S, Bevelander G, Tiamsic T: Growth inhibition of prematures receiving tetracycline. Am J Dis Child 105:453–461, 1963.
33. Dern RJ, Beutler E, Alving AS: Hemolytic effect of primaquine. II. The natural course of the hemolytic anemia and the mechanism of its self-limited character. J Lab Clin Med 4:171–176, 1954.
33a. De Troyer A, Demanet JC: Correction of antidiuresis by demeclocycline. N Engl J Med 293:915–918, 1975.
34. de Weck AL, Blum G: Recent clinical and immunological aspects of penicillin allergy. Int Arch Allergy Appl Immunol 27:221–256, 1965.
35. de Weck AL, Girard JP: Specific inhibition of allergic reactions to penicillin in man by a monovalent hapten. Int Arch Allergy Appl Immunol 42:798–815, 1972.
36. Dietschy JM, Siperstein M: Cholesterol synthesis by the gastrointestinal tract: localization and mechanisms of control. J Clin Invest 44:1311–1327, 1965.
37. Dobbins WO III, Herrero BA, Mansbach CM: Morphologic alterations associated with neomycin induced malabsorption. Am J Med Sci 255:63–77, 1968.
38. Douglas JB, Healy JK: Nephrotoxic effects of amphotericin B, including renal tubular acidosis. Am J Med 46:154–162, 1969.
39. Ellis FG: Acute polyneuritis after nitrofurantoin therapy. Lancet 2:1136–1138, 1962.
40. Feinberg JG: Experimental studies on penicillin allergy. In Penicillin Allergy. Edited by Stewart GT, McGovern JP. Springfield, Ill., Charles C Thomas, 1970, pp. 90–110.
41. Finegold SM, Miller LG, Posnick D, et al: Nalidixic acid: clinical and laboratory studies. Antimicrob Agents Chemother 189–197, 1966.
42. Fisher OD: Nalidixic acid and intracranial hypertension. Br Med J 3:370–371, 1967.
43. Friedmann I, Dadswell JV, Bird ES: Electron-microscope studies of the

neuroepithelium of the inner ear in guinea-pigs treated with neomycin. J Pathol Bacteriol 92:415–422, 1966.

44. Frimpter GW, Timpanelli AE, Eisenmenger WJ, et al: Reversible "Fanconi syndrome" caused by degraded tetracycline. JAMA 184:111–113, 1963.

45. Gaudefroy M, Viart P: Influence des antibiotiques sur la recrudescence actuelle des vaginités mycosiques. [Effects of antibiotics on the recurrence of fungal vaginitis.] Ann Biol Clin 13:113–120, 1955.

46. Glynn KP, Cafaro AF, Fowler CW, et al: False elevations of serum glutamic-oxalacetic transaminase due to para-aminosalicylic acid. Ann Intern Med 72:525–527, 1970.

47. Gralnick HR, McGinniss M, Elton W, et al: Hemolytic anemia associated with cephalothin. JAMA 217:1193–1197, 1971.

48. Green GR: Antibiotic therapy in patients with a history of penicillin allergy. In Penicillin Allergy. Edited by Stewart GT, McGovern JP. Springfield, Ill., Charles C Thomas, 1970, pp. 162–175.

49. Green RL, Lewis JE, Kraus SJ, et al: Elevated plasma procaine concentrations after administration of procaine penicillin G. N Engl J Med 291:223–226, 1974.

50. Grossman ER, Walchek A, Freedman H: Tetracyclines and permanent teeth: the relation between dose and tooth color. Pediatrics 47:567–570, 1971.

51. Gupta S, Grieco MH, Siegel I: Suppression of T-lymphocyte rosettes by rifampin. Ann Intern Med 82:484–488, 1975.

52. Gutnick MJ, Prince DA: Penicillinase and the convulsant action of penicillin. Neurology (Minneap) 21:759–764, 1971.

53. Hailey FJ, Glascock HW Jr, Hewitt WF: Pleuropneumonic reactions to nitrofurantoin. N Engl J Med 281:1087–1090, 1969.

54. Handbook of Antimicrobial Therapy. The Medical Letter on Drugs and Therapeutics 14(2):16–17, 1972.

55. Hardison WG, Rosenberg IH: The effect of neomycin on bile salt metabolism and fat digestion in man. J Lab Clin Med 74:564–573, 1969.

56. Hoffbrand BI, Stewart JD: Carbenicillin and hypokalaemia. Br Med J 4:746, 1970.

57. Hoffman TA, Cestero R, Bullock WE: Pharmacodynamics of carbenicillin in hepatic and renal failure. Ann Intern Med 73:173–178, 1970.

58. Hulme B, Reeves DS: Leucopenia associated with trimethoprim-sulphamethoxazole after renal transplantation. Br Med J 3:610–612, 1971.

59. Iinuma T, Mizukoshi O, Daly JF: Possible effects of various ototoxic drugs upon the ATP-hydrolyzing system in the stria vascularis and spiral ligament of the guinea pig. Laryngoscope 77:159–170, 1967.

60. Jick H, Slone D, et al: Excess of ampicillin rashes associated with allopurinol or hyperuricemia. N Engl J Med 286:505–508, 1972.

61. Johanson WG, Pierce AK, Sanford JP: Changing pharyngeal bacterial flora of hospitalized patients. Emergence of gram-negative bacilli. N Engl J Med 281:1137–1140, 1969.

62. Kahn SB, Fein SA, Brodsky I: Effects of trimethoprim on folate metabolism in man. Clin Pharmacol Ther 9:550–560, 1968.

63. Keefer CS, Hewitt WL: Therapeutic Value of Streptomycin; A Study of 3000 Cases. Ann Arbor, Edwards Bros., 1948.

64. Kelly DR, Nilo ER, Berggren RB: Brief recording: deafness after topical neomycin wound irrigation. N Engl J Med 280:1338–1339, 1969.

65. Koch-Weser J, Gilmore EB: Benign intracranial hypertension in an adult after tetracycline therapy. JAMA 200:345–347, 1967.

66. Koch-Weser J, Sidel VW, Federman EB, et al: Adverse effects of sodium colistimethate. Manifestations and specific reaction rates during 317 courses of therapy. Ann Intern Med 72:857–868, 1970.

67. Kosek JC, Mazze RI, Cousins MJ: Nephrotoxicity of gentamicin. J Lab Invest 30:48–57, 1974.

68. Kutti J, Weinfield A: The frequency of thrombocytopenia in patients with heart disease treated with oral diuretics. Acta Med Scand 183:245–250, 1968.

69. La Du BN:Pharmacogenetics: defective enzymes in relation to reactions to drugs. Annu Rev Med 23:453–468, 1972.

70. Lal S, Singhal SN, Burley DM, et al: Effect of rifampicin and isoniazid on liver function. Br Med J 1:148–150, 1972.

71. Leach W: Ototoxicity of neomycin and other antibiotics. J Laryngol 76:774–790, 1962.

72. Levine BB: Antigenicity and cross-reactivity of penicillins and cephalosporins. J Infect Dis 128:Suppl:S364–366, 1973.
73. Levine BB: Induction of IgE antibody response. In The Biological Role of the Immunoglobulin E System. Edited by Ishizaka K, Dayton D. Washington, D.C., US Dept HEW, 1972, pp. 81–148.
74. Levine BB: Skin rashes with penicillin therapy: current management. N Engl J Med 286:42–43, 1972.
75. Levine BB, Redmond AP: Immunochemical mechanisms of penicillin induced Coombs positivity and hemolytic anemia in man. Int Arch Allergy 31:594–606, 1967.
76. Levine BB, Redmond AP, Fellner MJ, et al: Penicillin allergy and the heterogeneous immune responses of man to benzylpenicillin. J Clin Invest 45:1895–1906, 1966.
77. Levine BB, Redmond AP, Voss HE, et al: Prediction of penicillin allergy by immunological tests. Ann NY Acad Sci 145:298–309, 1967.
78. Levine BB, Zolov DM: Prediction of penicillin allergy by immunological tests. J Allergy 43:231–244, 1969 (April).
79. Levine PH, Regelson W, Holland JF: Chloramphenicol-associated encephalopathy. Clin Pharmacol Ther 11:194–199, 1970.
80. Lindesmith LA, Baines RD Jr, Bigelow DB, et al: Reversible respiratory paralysis associated with polymyxin therapy. Ann Intern Med 68:318–327, 1968.
81. Lindholm T: Electromyographic changes after nitrofurantoin (Furadantin) therapy in nonuremic patients. Neurology (Minneap) 17:1017–1020, 1967.
82. Lundquist PG, Wersäll J: The ototoxic effect of gentamicin—an electron microscopical study. In Gentamicin: First International Symposium. Lucerne, Switzerland, Essex Chimie Ag, 1967, pp. 26–46.
83. Maddrey W, Boitnott JK: Isoniazid hepatitis. Ann Intern Med 79:1–12, 1973.
84. Maroon JC, Mealy J Jr: Benign intracranial hypertension. Sequel to tetracycline therapy in a child. JAMA 216:1479–1480, 1971.
85. Martelo OJ, Manyon DR, Smith US: Chloramphenicol and bone marrow mitochondria. J Lab Clin Med 74:927–940, 1969.
86. Masterton G, Schofield CB: Letter: Side-effects of minocycline hydrochloride. Lancet 2(7889):1139, 1974.
87. Matz GJ, Wallace TH, Ward PH: The ototoxicity of kanamycin. Laryngoscope 75:1690–1698, 1965.
88. McClure PD, Casserly JG, Monsier C, et al: Carbenicillin-induced bleeding disorder. Lancet 2:1307–1308, 1970.
89. McCurdy DK, Frederic M, Elkington JR: Renal tubular acidosis due to amphotericin B. N Engl J Med 278:124–130, 1968.
90. McLaughlin JE, Reeves DS: Clinical and laboratory evidence for inactivation of gentamicin by carbenicillin. Lancet 1:261–264, 1971.
91. Meyers RM: Ototoxic effects of gentamicin. Arch Otolaryngol (Chicago) 92:160–162, 1970.
92. Mitus WJ, Coleman N: In vitro effect of chloramphenicol on chromosomes. Blood 35:689–694, 1970.
93. Morris JS: Nitrofurantoin and peripheral neuropathy with megaloblastic anemia. J Neurol Neurosurg Psychiat 29:224–228, 1966.
94. Nagao T, Mauer AM: Concordance of drug-induced aplastic anemia in identical twins. N Engl J Med 281:7–11, 1969.
95. Neuvonen PJ, Penttila O: Interaction between doxycycline and barbiturates. Br Med J 1:535–536, 1974.
96. Nicol CS, Oriel JD: Letter: Minocycline: Possible vestibular side-effects. Lancet 2(7891):1260, 1974.
97. Noone P, Pattison JR: Therapeutic implications of interaction of gentamicin and penicillins. Lancet 2:575–578, 1971.
98. Nordstrom L, Banck G, Belfrage S, et al: Prospective study of the ototoxicity of gentamicin. Acta Pathol Microbiol Scand [B] 241:Suppl:58–66, 1973.
99. Penttila O, Neuvonen PJ, Aho K, et al: Interaction between doxycycline and some antiepileptic drugs. Br Med J 2:470–472, 1974.
100. Powell SJ: The cardiotoxicity of systemic amebicides. A comparative electrocardiographic study. Am J Trop Med 16:447–450, 1967.
101. Price D, Graham DI: Effects of large doses of colistin sulfomethate sodium on renal function. Br Med J 4:525–527, 1970.
102. Pujet J, Homberg J, Decroix G: Sensitivity to rifampicin: incidence, mechanism, and prevention. Br Med J 2:415–418, 1974.

103. Ream CR: Respiratory and cardiac arrest after intravenous administration of kanamycin with reversal of toxic effects by neostigmine. Ann Intern Med 59:384–387, 1963.

104. Riff LJ, Jackson GG: Laboratory and clinical conditions for gentamicin inactivation by carbenicillin. Arch Intern Med 130:887–891, 1972.

105. Roelsen E: Polyneuritis after nitrofurantoin (Furadantin) therapy. A survey and report of two new cases. Acta Med Scand 175:145–154, 1964.

106. Rollo IM: Miscellaneous drugs used in the treatment of protozoal infections. In The Pharmacological Basis of Therapeutics, Ed. 4. New York, The Macmillan Co., 1970, pp. 1144–1153.

107. Rosenow EC III, DeRemee RA, Dines DE: Chronic nitrofurantoin pulmonary reaction. Report of 5 cases. N Engl J Med 279:1258–1262, 1968.

108. Rudolph AH, Price EV: Penicillin reactions among patients in venereal disease clinics. A national survey. JAMA 223:499–501, 1973.

109. Sabath LD, Gerstein DA, Finland M: Serum glutamic oxalacetic transaminase. False elevations during administration of erythromycin. N Engl J Med 279:1137–1139, 1968.

110. Saslaw S: Demethylchlortetracycline phototoxicity. N Engl J Med 264:1301–1302, 1961.

111. Scholand JF, Tennenbaum JI, Cerilli GJ: Anaphylaxis to cephalothin in a patient allergic to penicillin. JAMA 206:130–132, 1968.

112. Schultz JC, Adamson JS Jr, Workman WW, et al: Fatal liver disease after intravenous administration of tetracycline in high dosage. N Engl J Med 269:999–1004, 1963.

113. Seamans KB, Gloor P, Dobell RAR, et al: Penicillin-induced seizures during cardiopulmonary bypass. A clinical and electroencephalographic study. N Engl J Med 278:861–868, 1968.

114. Sheldon WH, Heyman A: Morphologic changes in syphilitic lesions during Jarisch-Herxheimer reaction. Am J Syph Gonor Ven Dis 33:213–224, 1949.

115. Shulman NR: Mechanism of blood cell destruction in individuals sensitized to foreign antigens. Trans Assoc Am Physicians 76:72–83, 1963.

116. Silverblatt F, Harrison WO, Turck M: Nephrotoxicity of cephalosporin antibiotics in experimental animals. J Infect Dis 128:Suppl:S367–377, 1973.

117. Singer I, Rotenberg D: Demeclocycline-induced nephrogenic diabetes insipidus. In-vivo and in-vitro studies. Ann Intern Med 79:679–683, 1973.

118. Solomon P: Oral moniliasis complicating combined broad-spectrum antibiotic and antifungal therapy. N Engl J Med 265:847–848, 1961.

119. Spink WW, Braude AI, Castaneda MR, et al: Aureomycin therapy in human brucellosis due to Brucella melitensis. JAMA 138:1145–1148, 1948.

120. Stewart GT: Hypersensitivity and toxicity of the beta-lactam antibiotics. Postgrad Med J 43:Suppl:31–36, 1967.

121. Tedesco FJ, Stanley RJ, Alpers DH: Diagnostic features of clindamycin-associated pseudomembranous colitis. N Engl J Med 290:841–843, 1974.

122. Tolman KG, Sannella JJ, Freston JW: Chemical structure of erythromycin and hepatotoxicity. Ann Intern Med 81:58–60, 1974.

123. Verhagen AR: Photosensitivity due to chlortetracycline. Dermatologica (Basel) 130:439–445, 1965.

124. Voss HE, Redmond AP, Levine BB: Clinical detection of the potential allergic reactor to penicillin by immunologic tests. JAMA 196:679–683, 1966.

125. Warner WA, Sanders E: Neuromuscular blockade associated with gentamicin therapy. JAMA 215:1153–1154, 1971.

126. Wemambu SN, Turk JL, Walters MF, et al: Erythema nodosum leprosum: a clinical manifestation of the arthus phenomenon. Lancet 2:933–935, 1969.

127. Whitman EN: Effects in man of prolonged administration of trimethoprim and sulfisoxazole. Postgrad Med J 45:Suppl:46–51, 1969.

128. Wilfert JN, Burke JP, Bloomer HA, et al: Renal insufficiency associated with gentamicin therapy. J Infect Dis 124:Suppl:148–153, 1971.

129. Williams DN, Laughlin LW, Lee Y: Minocycline: possible vestibular side-effects. Lancet 2:744–746, 1974.

130. Yunis AA, Smith US, Restrepo A: Reversible bone marrow suppression from chloramphenicol. A consequence of mitochondrial injury. Arch Intern Med (Chicago) 126:272–275, 1970.

131. Zauder HL, Barton N, Bennett EJ, et al: Colistimethate as a cause of postoperative apnoea. Canad Anaesth Soc J 13:607–610, 1966.

132. Zelickson AS: Phototoxic reaction with nalidixic acid. JAMA 190:556–557, 1964.

CHAPTER 7

TREATMENT

Treatment of infection is based on the principles of chemotherapy discussed in the first six chapters. The objective is to get enough drug to the infecting organisms to inhibit or kill them without toxicity for the patient. The following treatment schedules are for adults and take into account the absorption, distribution, and excretion of the drug, its potential toxicity, and the nature and location of the infection. Alternates are given for patients who cannot tolerate the treatment of choice. If no duration is stated, treatment must be continued until no further signs of disease are evident.

UPPER RESPIRATORY TRACT
AND ORAL INFECTIONS

Pharyngitis and Tonsillitis

TREATMENT OF CHOICE	ALTERNATE
Group A streptococcus[67]	
Benzathine penicillin, 1,200,000 units intramuscularly, or penicillin V, 500 mg orally 4 times daily for 10 days	Erythromycin or cephalexin, 250 mg orally 4 times daily for 10 days
C. diphtheriae (carrier state)[12, 76]	
Erythromycin, 500 mg orally 4 times daily for 14 days	Procaine penicillin, 600,000 units intramuscularly daily for 14 days, or benzathine penicillin, 1,200,000 units intramuscularly

148

Pharyngitis and Tonsillitis (Continued)

TREATMENT OF CHOICE	ALTERNATE

N. gonorrhoeae

1 injection procaine penicillin, 4,800,000 units intramuscularly, plus 1 oral dose probenecid 1 gm | Tetracycline HCl, 1.5 gm orally 4 times daily for 4 days (total 9.5 gm)

Sinusitis and Otitis Media

Group A streptococcus

Penicillin V, 500 mg orally 4 times daily | Tetracycline or cephalexin 250 mg orally every 4 hours for 7–10 days

Pneumococcus

Penicillin V, 500 mg orally 4 times daily for 10 days | Tetracycline or cephalexin, 500 mg orally 4 times daily for 7–10 days

S. aureus (penicillinase-negative)

Penicillin V, 500 mg orally 4 times daily for 10 days | Cephalexin, 500 mg, plus probenecid, 0.5 gm orally 4 times daily for 10 days

S. aureus (penicillinase-positive)

Dicloxacillin or oxacillin, 500 mg orally 4 times daily for 10 days | Cephalexin, 500 mg, plus probenecid, 0.5 gm orally 4 times daily for 10 days

Anaerobic streptococcus

Buffered penicillin G, 400,000 units orally, plus probenecid, 0.5 gm orally 4 times daily | Cephalexin, 500 mg orally 4 times daily for 10 days

Bacteroides oralis

Buffered penicillin G, 400,000 units orally, plus probenecid, 0.5 gm orally 4 times daily | Cephalexin, 500 mg orally 4 times daily for 10 days

Epiglottitis

H. influenzae

Chloramphenicol, 1.0 gm intravenously every 6 hours until clinically arrested and sensitivities known | Penicillin G, 1,000,000 units intravenously every 4 hours, plus kanamycin, 0.5 gm every 6 hours until clinically arrested and sensitivities known

Ludwig's Angina

TREATMENT OF CHOICE	ALTERNATE
Group A streptococcus	
Penicillin G, 500,000 units intravenously every 3 hours, or procaine penicillin, 1,000,000 units intramuscularly every 8 hours	Cephalothin, 0.5 gm intravenously every 4 hours, or erythromycin lactobionate, 0.2 gm intravenously every 4 hours

Vincent's Infections

Vincent's angina (acute fusospirochetal pharyngitis): fusobacteria and oral spirochetes

Procaine penicillin, 600,000 units intramuscularly twice daily	Tetracycline, 250 mg orally every 4 hours

Vincent's stomatitis (trench mouth)

Procaine penicillin, 600,000 units intramuscularly twice daily for 3–7 days, or metronidazole, 200 mg 3 times daily for 3–7 days[25, 38]	Tetracycline, 250 mg orally every 4 hours

Actinomycosis of the Jaw

A. israelii

Penicillin G, 500,000 units intravenously every 3 hours until clinical cure; then tetracycline, 500 mg orally every 8 hours for 14 days	Tetracycline, 500 mg orally every 8 hours until 2 weeks after clinical cure

Phycomycosis

Phycomycosis of turbinate and palate: *Rhizopus oryzae* and other *Mucorales*

Amphotericin B, 50–70 mg intravenously daily (total course 2.0–2.5 gm)	None

African nasal phycomycosis: *Entomophthora coronata*

Potassium iodide, 10 drops orally 3 times daily to start and gradually increased to tolerance	Amphotericin B, 30–50 mg intravenously daily

Thrush of the Mouth

TREATMENT OF CHOICE ALTERNATE

C. albicans

Nystatin oral solution, 2 ml (200,000 units per ml) as mouthwash 4 times daily after meals

Amphotericin B, 2 ml (80 mg per ml) as mouthwash 4 times daily after meals

Treponematoses

Bejel (mucous patches of mouth, palate, and larynx): *Treponema pallidum* II

Benzathine penicillin, 1,200,000 units intramuscularly in 1 dose

Procaine penicillin in 2% aluminum monostearate, 1,200,000 units intramuscularly in 1 dose

Gangosa (nasopalatal yaws): *Treponema pertenue*

Procaine penicillin in 2% aluminum monostearate, 2,400,000 units intramuscularly in 1 dose[50]

Oxytetracycline or chlortetracycline, 500 mg orally every 6 hours for 10 days

Syphilis (oral chancre [primary] or mucous patches [secondary]): *T. pallidum*

Procaine penicillin, 600,000 units intramuscularly per day for 10 days; benzathine penicillin, 2,400,000 units in 1 dose for chancre and in 2 doses (the second after 1 week) for mucous patches[88]

Erythromycin or tetracycline, 500 mg orally every 6 hours for 10–14 days

Herpes Stomatitis

Herpes simplex I

5% idoxuridine in Orabase[53] None

The objective of treatment varies with the infection. In streptococcal pharyngitis the objective is not only cure of the sore throat but also prevention of rheumatic fever. Duration of treatment may be the key; 10 days are needed to eliminate the streptococcus from the throat of most patients.[28] One injection of benzathine penicillin produces effective levels for twice that period. In diphtheria, on the other hand, antibiotics cannot cure the disease because they cannot neutralize the effects of diphtheria toxin. Treatment can only eliminate the diphtheria carrier state. Erythromycin is the best available drug for this purpose.[12]

In sinusitis, as in other purulent conditions, drainage may be as important as antibiotics. Penicillin and tetracycline are the drugs of choice when the organisms are sensitive because they enter the sinuses in therapeutic concentrations. In the occasional sinus infection due to *S. aureus* resistant to tetracycline, cephalexin is recommended for patients with a history of penicillin allergy. Probenecid should be used to assure adequate levels, because serum levels with 500 mg cephalexin are only twice the minimal inhibitory concentration (MIC) for S. aureus.

Chloramphenicol is listed as the drug of choice for H. influenzae epiglottitis because strains resistant to penicillin and ampicillin have developed.[61, 97] Since epiglottitis is a life-threatening fulminant illness the risk of resistance, even though small, cannot be taken. The alternative is to cover the risk of resistance to penicillin by giving it in conjunction with kanamycin. For this reason the penicillin-kanamycin combination is given as second choice for patients who cannot be given chloramphenicol because of allergy or hematologic depression. The dose of kanamycin listed will give peak serum levels five to eight times the MIC for H. influenzae.

Two instances in which penicillin may be disputed as the drug of choice are the anaerobic infections caused by Vincent's organisms and by A. israelii. Metronidazole is considered by some to be superior to penicillin in Vincent's infections, and the tetracyclines have been used successfully in patients with actinomycosis who failed to respond to penicillin.[66, 77] With either penicillin or tetracycline, treatment of actinomycosis should be

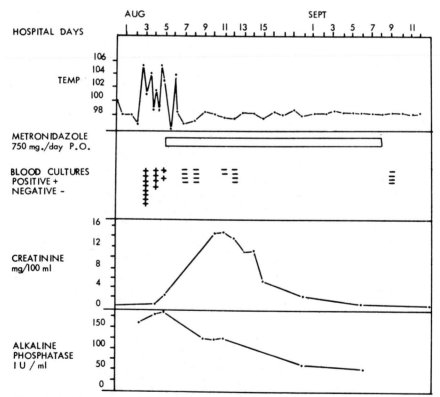

Figure 7–1. Cure of *Fusobacterium necrophorum* septicemia with metronidazole. (From Tally FP, Sutter VL, Finegold SM: Metronidazole versus anaerobes. Calif Med *117*:23, 1972.)

continued for several weeks after the patient appears cured because relapses occur from inapparent foci of infection. The success of metronidazole in Vincent's infections and its activity *in vitro* against anaerobes have led to its use in other anaerobic infections, but clinical experience is too limited to draw any conclusions about its general efficacy[95] (Fig. 7–1).

PULMONARY INFECTIONS

Pneumonia

TREATMENT OF CHOICE	ALTERNATE
Pneumococcus and group A streptococcus	
Procaine penicillin, 600,000 units intramuscularly every 12 hours for 7 days[15]	Cefazolin, 0.5 gm intramuscularly every 12 hours for 7 days,[99] or cephalexin, 500 mg orally every 6 hours
Meningococcus	
Procaine penicillin 600,000 units intramuscularly every 12 hours for 7 days	Chloramphenicol, 500 mg orally or 1.0 gm intravenously every 6 hours
M. pneumoniae	
Tetracycline, 500 mg orally 3 times daily for 5 days	Erythromycin stearate, 500 mg orally 3 times daily for 5 days
Chlamydia psittaci (ornithosis)	
Tetracycline, 500 mg orally 4 times daily for 14 days	Penicillin G, 1,000,000 units intravenously every 4 hours for 10 to 14 days
Coxiella burnetii (Q fever)	
Tetracycline, 500 mg orally 4 times daily for 14 days	Chloramphenicol, 500 mg orally 4 times daily for 14 days
Pneumocystis carinii	
Pentamidine isethionate, 300 mg intramuscularly daily for 12 days[102]	Pyrimethamine, 25 mg orally twice daily, and sulfadiazine, 1 gm orally 4 times daily (Fig. 7–2)
Toxoplasma gondii	
Pyrimethamine, 50 mg daily for 3 days; then 25 mg daily plus trisulfapyrimidines, 1.0 gm orally 4 times daily	None

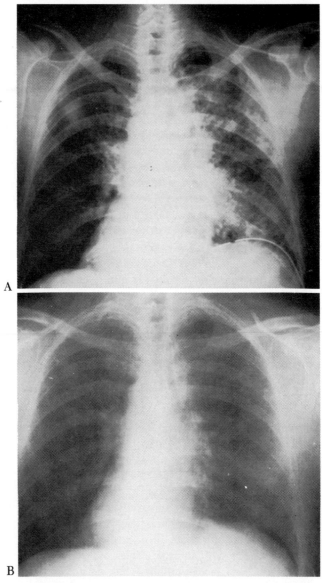

Figure 7–2. Treatment of *Pneumocystis carinii* pneumonia. *A,* Chest x-ray taken the day before institution of pyrimethamine and sulfadiazine shows bilateral infiltrates. *B,* Chest x-ray taken two weeks after completion of pyrimethamine and sulfadiazine therapy. The infiltrates have cleared, leaving a mild degree of pulmonary fibrosis. (From Kirby HB, Kenamore B, Guckian JC: *Pneumocystis carinii* pneumonia treated with pyrimethamine and sulfadiazine. Ann Intern Med 75:507, 1971.)

Pneumonia and Lung Abscess

TREATMENT OF CHOICE	ALTERNATE

S. *aureus* (penicillinase-negative)
 Penicillin G, 2,000,000 units every 6 hours intravenously until cure | Cefazolin, 1 gm every 6 hours intramuscularly or intravenously

S. *aureus* (penicillinase-positive)
 Methicillin, 1.0 gm intravenously every 3 hours | Cefazolin, 1 gm every 6 hours intramuscularly or intravenously

H. *influenzae*
 Penicillin G, 1,000,000 units intravenously every 6 hours, or ampicillin, 0.5 gm intravenously every 6 hours | Chloramphenicol, 500 mg orally every 4 hours or 1.0 gm intravenously every 6 hours

Anaerobic streptococcus
 Penicillin G, 1,000,000 units intravenously every 6 hours | Clindamycin, 300 mg intravenously every 4 hours or 450 mg orally every 6 hours

P. *aeruginosa*
 Carbenicillin, 2.0 gm intravenously every 2 hours, plus gentamicin, 80 mg intravenously every 8 hours[92] | Polymyxin B or colistin, 80 mg intramuscularly every 8 hours

K. *pneumoniae*
 Gentamicin, 80 mg intravenously 3 times daily, plus chloramphenicol succinate, 1.0 gm intravenously every 6 hours | Kanamycin, 0.5 gm intramuscularly every 6 hours, plus chloramphenicol succinate, 1.0 gm intravenously every 6 hours

P. *pseudomallei*
 Tetracycline, 0.5 gm every 4 hours, plus sulfisoxazole, 1.0 gm orally every 6 hours | Chloramphenicol, 0.5 gm every 3 hours, plus sulfisoxazole, 1.0 gm orally every 6 hours

Yersinia pestis
 Streptomycin, 0.5 gm intramuscularly every 6 hours for 5 days, plus tetracycline, 500 mg orally every 6 hours for 10 days | Streptomycin, 0.5 gm intramuscularly every 6 hours for 5 days, plus chloramphenicol, 500 mg orally 4 times daily for 10 days

Pneumonia and Lung Abscess *(Continued)*

TREATMENT OF CHOICE	ALTERNATE

Francisella tularensis
    Streptomycin, 0.5 gm intramuscularly every 6 hours for 3 days, then 0.5 gm every 8 hours for 3 days[78]

Tetracycline or chloramphenicol, 500 mg orally every 4 hours for 10 days[106]

A. israelii
    See treatment of actinomycosis of the jaw (p. 150)

N. asteroides
    Trisulfapyrimidines, 500 mg (167 mg each of sulfadiazine, sulfamerazine, and sulfamethazine), 2 tablets orally every 2 hours[41]

Cycloserine, 250 mg orally twice daily, or minocycline, 200 mg orally twice daily

M. tuberculosis
    Isoniazid, 300 mg, plus rifampin, 600 mg orally daily

Isoniazid, 300 mg, plus ethambutol, 1.0 gm orally daily

M. kansasii and *M. intracellulare*
    Streptomycin, 0.5 gm intramuscularly, plus rifampin,[89] 600 mg orally, plus isoniazid, 300 mg orally daily

Isoniazid, 300 mg, rifampin, 600 mg, and ethambutol, 1.0 gm orally daily

Blastomyces dermatitidis[2]
    Amphotericin B, 40 mg intravenously every other day (total 1.6 gm)

5-Hydroxystilbamidine, 250 mg intravenously daily for 20–40 days

Paracoccidioides brasiliensis
    Amphotericin B, 40 mg intravenously every other day (total 1.6 gm)

Sulfadiazine, 1.0 gm every 4 hours

Histoplasma capsulatum[2]
    Amphotericin B, 40 mg intravenously every other day (total 2.0 gm)

None

Coccidioides immitis
    Amphotericin B, 50–70 mg intravenously every other day (total 2–2.5 gm)

None

Cryptococcus neoformans
    Amphotericin B, 40 mg intravenously every other day (total 1.6 gm)

Flucytosine, 2.0 gm orally every 6 hours

Pneumonia and Lung Abscess *(Continued)*

TREATMENT OF CHOICE   ALTERNATE

Aspergillus fumigatus (invasive)
Amphotericin B, 40 mg intrave-   None
nously daily until arrested

A. fumigatus (allergic)
Prednisone, 30 mg orally daily   None

The daily dose and duration of treatment of pneumonia with benzyl-penicillin are less for pneumococci than for penicillinase-negative staphylococci because staphylococcal pneumonia is frequently accompanied by staphylococcal endocarditis and by abscesses. In addition, staphylococci are two to three times less sensitive to penicillin than pneumococci. The reason for using higher prolonged doses of penicillin for endocarditis is discussed later. Larger doses in abscesses may be needed because staphylococci in leukocytes are protected from penicillin. Levels of penicillin that kill extracellular staphylococci do not prevent survival of staphylococci ingested by phagocytic cells.[74] Penicillin should be given in doses high enough to overcome this barrier to intracellular organisms and continued until bacteria are released from dead phagocytes.

Although ampicillin is usually regarded as superior to benzylpenicillin for *H. influenzae* infections, there is no basis for this choice in comparative clinical studies or sensitivity tests (see Chapter 3). Chloramphenicol is listed as an alternative drug for strains of *H. influenzae* that produce penicillinase. Penicillin is also listed as the drug of choice for anaerobic streptococcal infection of the lung even though anaerobic gram-negative bacilli and other anaerobes are involved. The most prominent of these are *Fusobacterium* and *Bacteroides*, but only *Bacteroides fragilis* is likely to be highly resistant to penicillin. Since penicillin is effective clinically in anaerobic lung infections,[1] it would seem that *B. fragilis* is either uncommon or unimportant in the pathogenesis of aspiration lung abscess, or that it cannot maintain infection if more virulent associated bacteria are destroyed by penicillin.

Combinations of drugs are given for the treatment of *Pseudomonas*, *Klebsiella*, and *Yersinia* (plague) infections of the lung. In *P. aeruginosa* infections, combined carbenicillin-gentamicin therapy offers potential synergism and covers the possibility of resistance to carbenicillin in a disease that can be too fulminating to risk incorrect antibiotics. The same is true for *K. pneumoniae*. In plague pneumonia, the second drug is used to *prevent* resistance to streptomycin. The same principle is behind the use of two drugs simultaneously in tuberculosis. Three drugs are used in *M. kansasii* and *M. intracellulare* infections on the basis of sensitivity tests and in order to gain net inhibition from the total that is not achieved by an individual drug. This additive effect seems to work out in successfully treated cases of *M. kansasii* infections but less often with *M. intracellulare*, which has too much innate resistance to all available drugs. For this reason surgical resection is usually necessary for *M. intracellulare*. Combinations of sulfonamides in nocardiosis are used for an entirely different reason. The object of mixing sulfonamides is to reduce the danger of crystallization in the urine without lowering the total sulfonamide dose. This is possible because the solubility in urine of each of the three sulfonamides is unaffected by the others.[68] Combinations of antibiotics, based on sensitivity testing, may be of value for nocardial infections that cannot be treated with sulfonamides. A combination of erythromycin and ampicillin is said to be synergistic against most strains of *N. asteroides in vitro* and has produced clinical improvement in pulmonary nocardiosis.[7]

In the pulmonary mycoses, amphotericin stands out as the drug of choice for most fungi and is seldom given with another antifungal drug. It is especially effective in North and South American blastomycosis, and in chronic or miliary histoplasmosis of the lung, but may also be of value in chronic cavitary coccidioidomycosis and in certain forms of cryptococcosis.[86] Amphotericin is disappointing in pulmonary aspergillosis because the fungi may be insensitive to the drug and inaccessible in the infarcted areas of the lung. In allergic bronchopulmonary aspergillosis, corticosteroids are curative. They suppress bronchial edema and secretions so that the fungus can be eliminated from the respiratory tract.[39] For patients who cannot take amphotericin B, sulfadiazine may be of temporary value in South American blastomycosis, but relapses may be expected after dramatic clinical response. In North American blastomycosis, hydroxystilbamidine is a good substitute for amphotericin and, with the exception of occasional fifth nerve injury, is much less toxic. Hydroxystilbamidine is ineffective, however, in South American blastomycosis. 5-Fluorocytosine is the only substitute available for pulmonary cryptococcosis and should be used if the yeast is sensitive. Unfortunately, cryptococci often become resistant to 5-fluorocytosine during treatment.

ABDOMINAL INFECTIONS

Enteritis

TREATMENT OF CHOICE	ALTERNATE
Typhoid fever (*S. typhosa*)	
Chloramphenicol, 1.0 gm orally every 6 hours until patient is afebrile, then 0.5 gm every 6 hours for 14 days, or ampicillin, 2.0 gm intravenously every 6 hours for 14 days (Fig. 7–3)	Trimethoprim, 160 mg, and sulfamethoxazole, 800 mg orally every 12 hours[93]
Typhoid carriers (normal gallbladders)	
Ampicillin, 1.5 gm, plus probenecid, 0.5 gm orally every 6 hours for 30 days[90]	Trimethoprim, 160 mg, and sulfamethoxazole, 800 mg orally twice daily for 90 days[84]

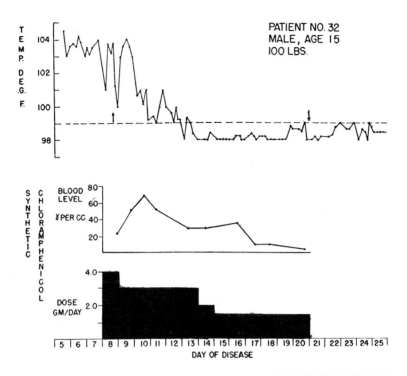

Figure 7–3. Response of typhoid fever to chloramphenicol. Fever characteristically returns to normal only after three to four days. (From Smadel JE, Bailey CA, Lewthwaite R: Synthetic and fermentation type chloramphenicol (chloromycetin) in typhoid fever: prevention of relapses by adequate treatment. Ann Intern Med 33:4, 1950.)

Enteritis (*Continued*)

TREATMENT OF CHOICE	ALTERNATE

Shigellosis
    Ampicillin, 1.0 gm 3 times daily orally for 3 days   Tetracycline, 2.5 gm orally in 1 dose

Cholera (*Vibrio cholerae*)
    Tetracycline, 0.5 gm orally every 6 hours,[42] or furazolidone, 200 mg orally every 6 hours for 2 days   Trimethoprim, 80 mg, and sulfamethoxazole, 400 mg orally every 6 hours[19] for 2 days

Yersinia enterocolitica and *Y. pseudotuberculosis*
    Streptomycin, 10 gm intramuscularly twice daily, or tetracycline, 0.5 gm orally every 6 hours for 4–6 days   Kanamycin, 1.0 gm intramuscularly twice daily, or ampicillin, 0.5 gm orally every 6 hours for 4–6 days

Enteritis (Continued)

TREATMENT OF CHOICE	ALTERNATE
Amebic dysentery (E. histolytica)	
Metronidazole, 750 mg orally 3 times daily for 10 days, or emetine HCl, 65 mg intramuscularly daily for 10 days, plus chloroquine, 250 mg orally twice daily for 14 days	Tetracycline, 0.5 gm orally 4 times daily for 10 days, plus chloroquine, 250 mg orally twice daily for 14 days
Giardiasis (Giardia lamblia)	
Metronidazole, 250 mg orally 3 times daily for 5 days	Atabrine, 100 mg orally 3 times daily for 5 days
Balantidiasis (Balantidium coli)	
Tetracycline, 0.5 gm orally 4 times daily for 10 days	Diodoquin, 650 mg orally 3 times daily for 20 days

Helminthiasis

Ascariasis (Ascaris lumbricoides)	
Piperazine citrate, 4.0 gm orally after breakfast for 2 days, or 1.0 gm via nasogastric tube every 24 hours for 6 days for intestinal obstruction	Pyrantel pamoate, 1.0 gm orally for 1 dose[11]
Strongyloidiasis (Strongyloides stercoralis)	
Thiabendazole, 1.5 gm orally twice daily for 2 days after meals	None
Hookworm (Necator americanus or Ancylostoma duodenale)	
Tetrachlorethylene, 5 ml orally for 1 dose	Bephenium hydroxynaphthoate, 5.0 gm orally for 1 dose for A. duodenale and for 3 days for N. americanus[107]
Trichuriasis (Trichuris trichiura)	
Thiabendazole, 1.5 gm orally twice daily for 2 days after meals	Mebendazole, 100 mg orally twice daily for 2 days
Cestodiasis (Taenia saginata, T. solium, and Hymenolepis nana)	
Niclosamide, 2.0 gm orally for 1 day[81]; same dosage for 5 days for H. nana	Paromomycin sulfate, 4.0 gm orally for 1 dose[104]
Schistosomiasis (Schistosoma mansoni)[32]	
Niridazole, 500 mg orally 3 times daily with meals	Sodium antimony tartrate, 10 ml (0.5% sol) intravenously day 1; 20 ml day 2; then 30 ml 4 times daily for 11 days; or stibophen (6.3% sol), 5 ml intramuscularly every other day for 16 days

Helminthiasis *(Continued)*

TREATMENT OF CHOICE   ALTERNATE

Schistosoma japonicum
  Sodium antimony tartrate as for
  S. mansoni

Diverticulitis

E. coli, Enterococcus, Peptostreptococcus, B. fragilis
  Chloramphenicol, 500 mg intra-   Doxycycline hyclate, 200 mg in-
  venously every 6 hours   travenously once daily

Cholecystitis and Cholangitis

E. coli, C. perfringens, Enterococcus, B. fragilis
  Ampicillin, 1.0 gm intravenously   Doxycycline hyclate, 200 mg in-
  every 6 hours, or tetracycline,   travenously once daily
  250 mg intravenously every 6
  hours

HEPATIC INFECTIONS

Liver Abscess

Pyogenic (pyelophlebitic): *B. fragilis*, anaerobic streptococci and *E. coli*
  Ampicillin, 2.0 gm intravenously   Tetracycline HCl, 250 mg every
  every 4 hours, plus clindamycin,   6 hours, or doxycycline hyclate,
  300 mg intravenously every 4   200 mg intravenously once daily
  hours; or chloramphenicol sodi-
  um succinate, 500 mg intravenously
  every 4 hours

E. histolytica
  Metronidazole, 750 mg orally 3   Emetine HCl, 65 mg intramuscu-
  times daily for 5 days   larly daily for 10 days, plus chlor-
                                     oquine, 250 mg orally twice daily
                                     for 28 days

Actinomycotic: *A. israelii*
  Tetracycline, 250 mg orally twice   Penicillin G, 1,000,000 units intra-
  daily, or doxycycline, 100 mg oral-   venously every 6 hours
  ly twice daily

Granulomatous Hepatitis

Miliary tuberculosis
  Isoniazid, 300 mg orally daily   Rifampin, 600 mg orally daily

Granulomatous Hepatitis (Continued)

Histoplasmosis, cryptococcosis, and coccidioidomycosis
  See treatment of pulmonary mycoses (p. 156)

C. burnetii
  See treatment of Q fever pneumonia (p. 153)

Hepatic Fascioliasis (Flukes)

Fasciola hepatica
  Emetine HCl, 65 mg intramuscu-   Bithionol, 200 mg orally every
  larly daily for 10 days   other day for 15 days, or chloro-
                                     quine phosphate, 250 mg orally
                                     3 times daily for 42 days

Clonorchis senensis
  Chloroquine phosphate, 250 mg   Bithionol, 200 mg orally every
  orally twice daily for 60–120 days other day for 15 days

Schistosomiasis
  See treatment of intestinal schistosomiasis (p. 160)

Leishmania donovani
  Antimony sodium gluconate, 600   Pentamidine isethionate, 200 mg
  mg intravenously daily for 10–14 intramuscularly daily for 15 days
  days

Spirochetal Hepatitis

Gummatous hepatitis: T. pallidum
  Aqueous procaine penicillin G,   Tetracycline or erythromycin, 0.5
  600,000 units intramuscularly daily gm orally every 4 hours for 30 days
  for 10–15 days, or benzathine
  penicillin G, 3,000,000 units intramuscularly once weekly for 3
  weeks

Leptospirosis (Leptospira interrogans, especially serogroup icterohemor-
rhagiae)
  Penicillin G, 1,000,000 units intra- Tetracycline, 0.5 gm orally 4 times
  venously 4 times daily for 7 days daily for 7 days

PERITONITIS

Primary: Pneumococcus and group A streptococcus
  See treatment of Pneumonia (p. 153)

PERITONITIS *(Continued)*

TREATMENT OF CHOICE	ALTERNATE

M. tuberculosis
Isoniazid, 300 mg orally daily   Rifampin, 600 mg orally daily

Secondary from bowel perforation: *E. coli, B. fragilis, S. fecalis, Peptostreptococcus*, fusobacteria

Chloramphenicol sodium succinate, 500 mg intravenously every 4 hours   Gentamicin, 70 mg intravenously every 6 hours, plus clindamycin, 300 mg intravenously every 4 hours, plus ampicillin, 20 gm intravenously every 6 hours

Secondary from female genitalia: clostridia, *E. coli, B. fragilis* and peptostreptococci
Same as bowel perforation

Gonococcus
Penicillin G, 1,000,000 units intravenously every 6 hours   Tetracycline HCl, 500 mg intravenously every 8 hours

Group A streptococcus
See treatment of primary peritonitis (p. 162)

Supportive therapy is sometimes more important than specific antimicrobials in gastrointestinal and other abdominal infections. Replacement of water and electrolytes is the only treatment usually needed for the dysentery of shigellosis, salmonellosis, cholera, *Vibrio parahemolytica* infection, clostridial enteritis, and invasive or enterotoxic *E. coli* diarrhea. With the exception of cholera (in which antibiotics reduce the number and size of stools) and severe *Shigella* infections, antibiotics are not indicated for treating bacterial dysentery. In fact, antibiotics actually interfere with the elimination of *Salmonella* from the bowel.[5] Drugs that retard gut motility, such as paregoric or the combination of dephenoxylate hydrochloride with atropine (Lomotil), should not be used in bacterial dysentery because they may prolong the fever and toxemia.[30]

Supportive therapy is equally important in peritonitis. Fluid and electrolyte replacement is crucial in the treatment of shock. Intubation and decompression must be used to alleviate vomiting or distention, and surgery is necessary to close or divert the perforation as soon as the patient's condition will allow. The antibiotics listed for peritonitis cover the important bacteria in patients who have not had a change in bowel flora from recent antibiotic therapy, or who develop peritonitis secondary to surgical wounds with staphylococci, *P. aeruginosa, K. pneumoniae, S. marcescens, E. aerogenes,* or *Proteus.* The treatment for staphylococcal, *Pseudomonas,* or *Klebsiella* peritonitis is the same as that described for pulmonary infections with those organisms. Infection with *P. mirabilis* will be covered adequately by the regimens listed for secondary peritonitis. Other *Proteus* species, *E. aerogenes*, and *S. marcescens* usually will respond to gentamicin plus carbenicillin. These antibiotic regimens are by no means absolute and must be guided by sensitivity tests. In patients with bowel flora sensitive to streptomycin, tetracycline, and ampicillin, these antibiotics in various combinations may be preferable to chloramphenicol with its risk of marrow depression.

Supportive treatment for localized infections varies with their locations. In diverticulitis, stool softeners and a liquid diet are required in mild cases. In other situations it may be necessary to drain abscesses and resect obstructing inflammatory masses or fistulae. In bacterial abscesses of the liver, subphrenic area, or pelvis, surgical drainage is more important than antibiotics. On the other hand, hepatic microabscesses occurring with pyelophlebitis or ascending cholangitis can be cured with antibiotics alone. The need for surgical drainage in amebic liver abscess is dubious since many cases have been cured with metronidazole.

Metronidazole has revolutionized the treatment of amebiasis, but it can only be given orally. Patients with severe amebic dysentery, who cannot take oral medication, are given emetine intramuscularly. Emetine and chloroquine are also needed for the occasional amebic liver abscess that appears resistant to metronidazole.[43]

Metronidazole is readily available commercially because it has been in use for treating vaginal trichomoniasis. Three other antiparasitic agents—niridazole, niclosamide, and bithionol—however, cannot be purchased in the United States and must be obtained from the Parasitic Diseases Drug Service (Parasitic Diseases Branch, Epidemiology Program, Center for Disease Control, Atlanta, Georgia 30333).

UROGENITAL INFECTIONS

Cystitis and Bladder Bacilluria[14]

TREATMENT OF CHOICE	ALTERNATE
E. coli	
Sulfisoxazole, 1.0 gm 3 times daily, or ampicillin, 250 mg orally 4 times daily for 5–8 days	Cephalexin, 250 mg 4 times daily, or tetracycline, 250 mg orally twice daily for 5–8 days
P. mirabilis	
Ampicillin, 250 mg 4 times daily for 5 days, or buffered penicillin G, 1.0 gm orally 4 times daily for 7 days	Cephalexin, 250 mg orally 4 times daily, or trimethoprim, 60 mg, plus sulfamethoxazole, 800 mg orally twice daily for 7 days

Cystitis and Bladder Bacilluria (Continued)

TREATMENT OF CHOICE ALTERNATE

P. aeruginosa, E. aerogenes, P. vulgaris

Indanyl carbenicillin, 1.0 gm, or tetracyline, 250 mg orally 4 times daily

Streptomycin, 0.5 gm, or gentamicin, 40 mg intramuscularly twice daily

K. pneumoniae

Cephalexin, 250 mg, or indanyl carbenicillin, 1.0 gm orally 4 times daily for 7 days

Trimethoprim, 160 mg, plus sulfamethoxazole, 800 mg orally twice daily, or gentamicin, 40 mg intramuscularly twice daily

S. fecalis

Ampicillin, 250 mg, or buffered penicillin G, 500 mg orally 4 times daily for 7 days

Tetracycline, 250 mg orally 4 times daily

Schistosoma hematobium

See treatment of Schistosoma mansoni infestation of bowel (p. 160)

Pyelonephritis[14]

E. coli

Ampicillin, 250 mg orally every 4 hours for 10 days; or streptomycin, 1.0 gm intramuscularly daily for 7 days, plus tetracycline, 250 mg orally twice daily for 21 days

Trimethoprim, 160 mg, plus sulfamethoxazole, 800 mg orally twice daily[16]

P. mirabilis

Ampicillin, 250 mg orally every 4 hours for 14 days, or penicillin G, 1,000,000 units intravenously every 6 hours for 7 days, then orally for 7 days

Cephalexin, 500 mg orally every 6 hours for 14 days, or trimethoprim, 160 mg, plus sulfamethoxazole orally twice daily[16]

P. aeruginosa

Carbenicillin, 1.0 gm intramuscularly daily for 10 days, or gentamicin, 40 mg intramuscularly 3 times daily for 7 days

Tetracycline, 250 mg orally every 6 hours, plus polymyxin B sulfate or sodium colistimethate, 40 mg intramuscularly 3 times daily

K. pneumoniae

Cefazolin, 1.0 gm intramuscularly twice daily for 7–10 days, or gentamicin, 40 mg intramuscularly 3 times daily

Cephalexin, 500 mg orally every 6 hours for 10 days, or trimethoprim, 160 mg, plus sulfamethoxazole, 800 mg orally 4 times daily for 14 days

Pyelonephritis (Continued)

TREATMENT OF CHOICE　　　　　　　ALTERNATE

S. fecalis
    Ampicillin, 500 mg orally every 6 hours, or streptomycin, 0.5 gm intramuscularly twice daily, plus buffered penicillin G, 500 mg orally every 6 hours for 10 days
    Gentamicin, 40 mg intramuscularly 3 times daily, plus ampicillin, 250 mg orally every 6 hours for 10 days

B. suis
    Tetracycline, 0.5 gm orally 4 times daily for 14 days
    Streptomycin, 1.0 gm intramuscularly daily, plus tetracycline, 0.5 gm orally 4 times daily for 10 days

C. albicans
    5-Fluorocytosine, 1.0 gm orally every 6 hours for 10 days
    Amphotericin B, 30–50 mg intravenously every other day

Aspergillosis (aspergilloma): A. fumigatus
    Amphotericin B, 40 mg intravenously every other day
    None

Cryptococcal pyelonephritis: Cryptococcus neoformans
    5-Fluorocytosine orally, 1.0 gm every 4 hours, or amphotericin B, 40 mg every other day for 40 days
    5-Fluorocytosine orally, 1.0 gm every 4 hours, plus amphotericin B, 20 mg every other day for 40 days

Histoplasmosis and blastomycosis of kidney
    See treatment of pulmonary histoplasmosis and blastomycosis (p. 156)

M. tuberculosis
    Isoniazid, 300 mg orally, plus ethambutol, 1.0 gm orally daily
    Streptomycin, 1.0 gm intramuscularly, plus para-aminosalicylic acid, 2.0 gm orally every 6 hours

A. israelii
    See treatment of actinomycosis of the jaw (p. 150)

Urethritis

N. gonorrhoeae[48]
    One injection of aqueous procaine penicillin G, 4,800,000 units intramuscularly (2,400,000 units in 2 sites), plus 1.0 gm probenecid, or 1 dose of ampicillin, 3.5 gm orally plus 1.0 gm probenecid orally
    Tetracycline HCl, 1.5 gm orally; then 0.5 gm orally 4 times daily for 4 days (total 9.5 gm) or 1 injection of spectinomycin HCl, 2.0 gm intramuscularly

Urethritis (Continued)

TREATMENT OF CHOICE   ALTERNATE

"Nonspecific" or postgonococcal (? T mycoplasma, ? *Mycoplasma hominis*, or ? *Chlamydia*)

Tetracycline, 0.5 gm 4 times daily for 7 days

Trimethoprim, 160 mg, and sulfamethoxazole, 800 mg orally twice daily for 7 days[17]

Trichomonas vaginalis

Metronidazole, 250 mg orally 3 times daily for 5 days

Nitrimidazine or metronidazole, 2.0 gm in a single dose

Cervicitis and Vulvovaginitis

N. gonorrhoeae

See treatment of urethritis

Trichomoniasis: *T. vaginalis*

See treatment of urethritis

Moniliasis: *C. albicans*

Nystatin tablets, 100,000 units in vaginal vault daily for 14 days

Candicidin tablets, 3 mg in vaginal vault twice daily for 14 days

Syphilis (chancre or mucous patches): *T. pallidum*

See treatment of oral syphilis (p. 151)

Lymphogranuloma venereum: *Chlamydia psittaci*[51]

Tetracycline, 0.5 gm orally 4 times daily for 14 days

Trisulfapyrimidines, 0.5 gm orally every 6 hours for 14 days

Granuloma inguinale: *Donovania granulomatis*

Tetracycline, 0.5 gm orally 4 times daily for 14–21 days

Erythromycin, 0.5 gm orally 4 times daily for 14–21 days

Genital herpes: *Herpesvirus hominis* II

0.5% idoxuridine ointment twice daily

Paint lesions with 40% idoxuridine in dimethyl sulfoxide 4 times daily for 3 days[52]

Endometritis and Salpingitis

N. gonorrhoeae

Penicillin G, 1,000,000 units intravenously every 6 hours for 10 days, or tetracycline, 1 dose of 1.5 gm orally, then 500 mg 4 times daily for 10 days

1 dose of ampicillin, 3.5 gm, plus probenecid 1.0 gm orally; then ampicillin, 500 mg orally 4 times daily for 10 days

Endometritis and Salpingitis (Continued)

TREATMENT OF CHOICE   ALTERNATE

M. tuberculosis
See treatment of pulmonary tuberculosis (p. 156)

Postabortal or postpartum: E. coli, B. fragilis, C. perfringens, enterococci, microaerophilic and anaerobic streptococci

| Chloramphenicol, 500 mg orally or intravenously every 3 hours | Ampicillin, 2.0 gm, and gentamicin, 80 mg intravenously every 6 hours, and clindamycin, 300 mg intravenously every 4 hours |

Actinomycosis
See treatment of actinomycosis of the jaw (p. 150)

Acute Prostatitis

E. coli, K. pneumoniae, P. mirabilis, P. aeruginosa, and E. aerogenes
See treatment of pyelonephritis (p. 165)

Chronic Prostatitis

S. aureus and S. fecalis

| Erythromycin, 0.5 gm 4 times daily | Trimethoprim, 160 mg, and sulfamethoxazole, 800 mg orally twice daily |

E. coli

| Doxycycline, 100 mg 4 times daily | Trimethoprim, 160 mg, and sulfamethoxazole, 800 mg orally twice daily |

Site of infection is probably the most important determinant of success in treating urinary infections. Bladder infections are easily eradicated, as a rule, by a short course of almost any drug to which the organism is sensitive at concentrations reached by the antibiotic in the urine rather than the blood (see Chapter 5). The main problem in bladder infections in women is recurrence. These recurring infections can be prevented by having the patient take 50 mg nitrofurantoin or apply an antibiotic ointment to the introitus before intercourse.[8] Pregnancy presents a special problem in the treatment of bladder infections because the normal dilatation of the upper collecting system increases susceptibility to pyelonephritis. Short courses of the antibiotics listed are as effective in eliminating bacilluria during pregnancy as is continuous treatment until term and virtually eliminate the risk of pyelonephritis.[103] E. coli is almost always responsible for bacilluria in pregnancy and is rarely resistant to drug therapy. If bacilluria recurs after the eight-day course, kidney infection is present and must be treated by continuous prophylaxis until term.

Pyelonephritis is usually more difficult to cure than bladder infections because of structural abnormalities or because the medulla is more difficult to rid of infection than the bladder. The first step in treating pyelonephritis is relief of obstruction, if present, because antibiotics cannot protect an obstructed kidney from destruction by acute infection. Acute pyelonephritis is usually caused by E. coli that are sensitive to most antimicrobial drugs in levels attainable in the urinary tract. Ampicillin is probably the most widely used treatment, but streptomycin is also effective. A low dose of tetracycline is given with streptomycin to prevent streptomycin-resistant mutants from overgrowing the bladder urine. Trimethoprim-sulfamethoxazole is at least as good as ampicillin in acute E. coli pyelonephritis and is better for recurrent or persistent urinary tract infections,[26] but thrombocytopenia may occur with the combination. Acute Proteus pyelonephritis responds to ampicillin or penicillin. Cure of Proteus infections is often difficult, however, because magnesium ammonium phosphate stones may be present.

Therapy of chronic pyelonephritis is less successful than of acute pyelonephritis. The chronic disease usually occurs because of stones, scars, and anatomic deformities that interfere with the ability of the drugs to eradicate the bacteria. If cure cannot be achieved, antimicrobials are given indefinitely in low dosage in order to suppress growth in the urine and prevent recurrence of symptoms. A similar problem is seen in men whose prostates are sites of persistent infection that cannot be eradicated by any drug. Bacteria from these prostates enter the urine and cause periodic E. coli infections with high fever and other systemic signs of pyelonephritis. Such attacks can be permanently prevented by continuous treatment with 250 mg ampicillin twice daily or small doses of other antibacterial drugs.[94]

Urinary infections in patients with indwelling catheters are best controlled by antibiotics introduced into the bladder through a triple lumen catheter. This permits a continuous rinse with a solution containing 40 mg neomycin or 20 mg polymyxin B in a liter of isotonic saline. This procedure may prevent bacteriuria and reduce the incidence of associated bacteremia by 75 per cent.[75] Good results are also obtained by using 0.25 per cent acetic acid for the bladder rinse instead of the antibiotics.[57]

The commonest cause of fungus infection of the kidney is Candida albicans. The heavy urinary excretion of 5-fluorocytosine produces remarkable reversal of severe renal moniliasis not seen with other therapy; it should be used for treating cryptococcal pyelonephritis as well. A few patients with aspergillosis of the kidney pelvis have improved after treatment with amphotericin B.

At least two antituberculosis drugs are required for treating urinary tuberculosis because resistant mutants grow well in the urine, and a second drug is necessary to inhibit them. It is reasonable to begin treatment with three drugs to assure the patient of at least two that are effective until sensitivities are known, and then to drop the third. Isoniazid, ethambutol, and streptomycin are probably the best suited pharmacologically for treating urinary tuberculosis because of their heavy excretion into the urine (see Tables 5–1 and 5–2). Rifampin, on the other hand, is excreted poorly into the urine and has not been proved to be of value in urinary tuberculosis.

With the exception of E. coli, the spectrum of bacteria involved in genital infections is entirely different from those in the urinary tract. The venereal agents responsible for communicable genital disease and the anaerobes that are prominent in endogenous genital infection almost never invade the bladder or kidney. Since they seldom exhibit the high degree of drug resistance found in the urinary enteric bacilli, definite treatment schedules can be formulated for genital infections. The gonococcus develops resistance to penicillin and tetracycline, but it is readily overcome by increasing the dosage. Either procaine penicillin or ampicillin with probenecid will cure most infections, and a course of tetracycline is reliable for those allergic to penicillins. The only problem with penicillin allergy in gonorrhea is encountered in pregnant women because tetracycline is damaging to the fetus. They should receive one dose of 0.5 gm erythromycin orally followed by 0.5 gm erythromycin four times daily for a total of 9.5 gm. Resistance to penicillin is also a problem with B. fragilis, but it is not overcome by increased dosage. Instead, chloramphenicol or clindamycin is recommended.

Pelvic anaerobic infections can be treated with chloramphenicol or clindamycin because these drugs are active against all the pelvic anaerobic bacteria, including B. fragilis. Infections with clostridia or anaerobic streptococci can be treated with penicillin as well. The patient with clostridial endometritis and myometritis should be treated by intravenous infusion of 20 million units of benzylpenicillin daily and by prompt removal of necrotic infected tissue by hysterectomy or curettage. She must also receive treatment for shock and renal failure. Debridement and drainage of pelvic abscesses are essential for successful antibiotic treatment of nonclostridial anaerobic pelvic infections.

Two of the more difficult genital infections to cure are chronic prostatitis and genital herpes. Acute prostatitis responds to the same treatment as urinary infections because the acute inflammatory response delivers the antibiotics to the gland. In chronic prostatitis, however, most antibiotics effective against the agents of prostatitis are unable to reach therapeutic levels in the gland for the reasons given in Chapter 5. Doxycycline may be an exception, however, and merits a trial before resorting to chronic suppressive therapy to prevent recurrent urinary infections.[36]

Inadequate penetration to the site of infection may also be the reason why herpes of the skin does not respond to topical idoxuridine, a drug that is of proved value in herpetic keratitis. Well-controlled studies have demonstrated that extragenital herpes of the skin does not respond to topical idoxuridine, but it is possible that some effect may occur on the thin skin of the genitalia. The claim is made that in many patients recurrences are fewer and of shorter duration if new lesions are painted with 40 per cent idoxuridine in DMSO (dimethyl sulfoxide) four times daily for three days.[53]

NEUROLOGIC INFECTIONS

Meningitis

Treatment of Choice	Alternate
Pneumococcus, meningococcus, group B streptococcus, S. aureus (penicillinase-negative), and C. perfringens	
Penicillin G, 2,000,000 units intravenously every 2 hours for 10 days	Chloramphenicol sodium succinate, 1.0 gm intravenously every 3 hours
S. aureus (penicillinase-positive)	
Methicillin or oxacillin, 1.0 gm intravenously every 2 hours	Chloramphenicol sodium succinate, 1.0 gm intravenously every 3 hours
P. mirabilis, H. influenzae, P. multocida, L. monocytogenes	
Ampicillin, 1.5 gm, or penicillin G, 2,000,000 units intravenously every 2 hours	Chloramphenicol sodium succinate, 1.0 gm intravenously every 3 hours
E. coli, Salmonella species	
Chloramphenicol sodium succinate, 1.0 gm intravenously every 3 hours	Ampicillin, 2.0 gm intravenously every 3 hours
K. pneumoniae	
Carbenicillin, 2.5 gm intravenously every 2 hours, plus gentamicin, 80 mg intravenously every 6 hours	Chloramphenicol sodium succinate, 1.0 gm intravenously every 3 hours
P. aeruginosa	
Carbenicillin, 2.5 gm intravenously every 2 hours, plus gentamicin, 80 mg intravenously every 6 hours	Gentamicin, 5.0 mg intrathecally, or polymyxin B, 2.0 mg intrathecally daily
B. abortus, B. suis, and B. melitensis	
Tetracycline, 0.5 gm orally 4 times daily	Chloramphenicol, 0.5 gm orally 4 times daily

Meningitis (Continued)

TREATMENT OF CHOICE	ALTERNATE

S. fecalis

Ampicillin, 1.5 gm, or penicillin G, 2,000,000 units intravenously every 2 hours, plus streptomycin, 1.0 gm twice daily intramuscularly

Ampicillin, 1.5 gm, or penicillin G, 2,000,000 units intravenously every 2 hours, plus gentamicin, 100 mg every 8 hours daily intravenously

M. tuberculosis

Isoniazid, 300 mg orally daily   None

Cryptococcosis: C. neoformans

5-Fluorocytosine, 2.0 gm orally every 6 hours, plus amphotericin B, 20 mg intravenously daily for 6 weeks, after initial amphotericin doses of 1.0 mg on day 1, 5 mg on day 2, 10 mg on day 3, and 15 mg on day 4[99a]

Amphotericin B, 40–60 mg intravenously every other day (total dose 3.0 gm), or amphotericin B, 0.5 mg intrathecally every other day, plus amphotericin B intravenously as above (for patients who cannot tolerate 5-fluorocytosine)

Coccidioidomycosis: C. immitis

Amphotericin B intravenously and intrathecally as for C. neoformans   None

Syphilitic meningitis: T. pallidum

Aqueous procaine penicillin, 600,000 units intramuscularly daily for 15 days

Tetracycline, 0.5 gm 4 times daily for 15 days

Cerebritis, Encephalitis, and Brain Abscess

Anaerobic streptococcus, B. fragilis, Fusobacterium, Actinomyces sp., and Hemophilus aphrophilus

Penicillin G, 2,000,000 units intravenously every 2 hours, plus chloramphenicol succinate, 1.0 gm intravenously every 3 hours

Cephalothin, 1.5 gm intravenously every 2 hours, plus chloramphenicol succinate, 1.0 gm intravenously every 3 hours

Rhizopus oryzae and other Mucorales

See treatment of phycomycosis of nasal turbinates (p. 150)

Nocardia asteroides

See treatment of pulmonary nocardiosis (p. 156)

General paresis and tabes dorsalis: T. pallidum

Aqueous procaine penicillin, 600,000 units intramuscularly daily for 15 days

Tetracycline, 0.5 gm orally 4 times daily for 15 days

Cerebritis, Encephalitis, and Brain Abscess (Continued)

TREATMENT OF CHOICE	ALTERNATE

Toxoplasma gondii
Pyrimethamine, 50 mg orally daily   None
for 3 days, then 25 mg orally, plus
trisulfapyrimidines, 1.0 gm orally
every 4 hours

Amebiasis: *Naegleria gruberi*   None
Amphotericin B, 1.0 mg intrathecally daily plus 60 mg intravenously
every other day

African sleeping sickness: *Trypanosoma gambiense* and *T. rhodesiense*
Melarsoprol (Mel B) (trivalent me-   Tryparsamide, 200 mg, plus sura-
larsen oxide and dimercaprol   min, 700 mg, given separately in-
[BAL]), 5 ml 3.6% sol in propyl-   travenously once every 5 days for
ene glycol intravenously daily for   a total of 12 injections; repeat in
4 days; repeat in 2 weeks   4 weeks

Spinal Epidural Abscess

S. aureus (penicillinase-negative)
Penicillin G, 1.0 gm intravenously   Cefazolin, 1.0 gm intramuscularly
every 2 hours   every 8 hours

S. aureus (penicillinase-positive)
Methicillin or oxacillin, 1.0 gm in-   Cefazolin, 1.0 gm intramuscularly
travenously every 2 hours   every 8 hours

Subdural Empyema

S. aureus
See treatment of spinal epidural abscess

Anaerobic streptococci, *B. fragilis, Fusobacterium*
See treatment of cerebritis

The two most important antibiotics for treating bacterial infections of the nervous system are the penicillins and chloramphenicol. The pneumococcus, aerobic streptococcus, meningococcus, penicillinase-negative staphylococcus, influenza bacillus, *Listeria*, anaerobic streptococcus, and *T. pallidum* are the major causes of nervous system infection, and all are sensitive to benzylpenicillin in concentrations that can be reached in the nervous system during infection (see Chapter 5). Two other penicillins, ampicillin and carbenicillin, can be used for the gram-negative bacilli that are not sensitive to benzylpenicillin. Because of its excellent penetration and wide antibacterial spectrum, chloramphenicol is the drug of choice for most bacterial infections of the meninges in patients who are allergic to penicillin, and for penicillin-resistant or ampicillin-resistant strains of *H. influenzae*.

Early treatment is important in all forms of intracranial infection but especially so in anaerobic infections of the brain.[47] The best results and lowest mortality are obtained by starting antibiotic treatment during the stage of cerebritis before it progresses to brain abscess and becomes a surgical problem. Severe headache and fever in combination with congenital heart disease, or chronic suppuration in the ear, paranasal sinuses, or chest should raise the strongest suspicion of bacterial encephalitis. Since most brain abscesses are caused by anaerobic or microaerophilic bacteria, combined penicillin and chloramphenicol can be relied on in the cerebritis stage. Subdural empyema and spinal epidural abscess also require immediate treatment, but surgical drainage is more important than antibiotic therapy. Antibiotics should be directed against anaerobes and staphylococci in subdural empyema, but only against staphylococci in spinal epidural abscess. Nearly all acute spinal epidural abscesses are caused by *S. aureus* and progress to fulminant spinal cord injury and paralysis within a few hours if the lesion is not decompressed surgically.

Intrathecal therapy is necessary occasionally for *Pseudomonas* and fungus infections. In *Pseudomonas aeruginosa* meningitis, enough carbenicillin and gentamicin may sometimes reach the infection to cure the infection, but more resistant strains of *Pseudomonas* may require intrathecal gentamicin. Systemic therapy with amphotericin B or 5-fluorocytosine may also cure some patients with cryptococcal meningitis, but in other cases it is necessary to give intrathecal amphotericin B because of relapse or severe impairment of renal function. All patients with coccidioidal meningitis require intrathecal amphotericin B, often for many years and sometimes for life. The duration of intrathecal injections in both conditions depends on the course of the illness. In cryptococcal meningitis sterility of the spinal fluid is the best end point for stopping treatment, but in coccidioidal meningitis the organism may not be recovered in culture even in untreated active cases. For this reason the clinical responses and the disappearance of cells, excess protein, and coccidioidal antibody are used as a measure of adequate therapy. Amphotericin may be given intrathecally by the lumbar route with considerable effectiveness in some cases of cryptococcal and coccidioidal meningitis, but others require intracisternal or intraventricular injections. Intracisternal injection is especially indicated in coccidioidal meningitis where the long-term introduction of amphotericin into the lumbar space causes arachnoiditis. Intracisternal injections are dangerous and require great skill, while intraventricular administration must be done through an Ommaya valve. This valve, which consists of a subcutaneous reservoir placed under the scalp and connected with the ventricle by a catheter, is dangerous because of superinfection and adhesions. A new approach has been developed to prevent lumbar arachnoiditis and to deliver the drug to the brain stem; it involves the use of a hyperbaric solution. Ten per cent dextrose in water is used as a hyperbaric solution for carrying amphotericin B away from the injection site to the basilar cistern by placing the patient in the Trendelenburg position.[3] This promising method is now under evaluation (Fig. 7–4).

Intrathecal therapy with amphotericin B is also recommended for the rare case of amebic meningoencephalitis caused by *Naegleria* trophozoites because the organism is sensitive to amphotericin. In fact, the only recovery on record of this fulminant disease has been in a patient' given amphotericin B.[18] Two other protozoal infections of the brain, toxoplasmosis and trypanosomiasis, are treated systemically. Pyrimethamine and sulfonamides are recommended for toxoplasma encephalitis because the combination seems to be effective in systemic toxoplasmosis and toxoplasmosis of the eye.[34] Six mg folinic acid daily is used to prevent the hematologic effects of folate deficiency induced by the pyrimethamine. The treatment of trypanosomal meningoencephalitis is better established than that of toxoplasma encephalitis. Melarsoprol (Mel B), a combination of trivalent melarsen oxide and dimercaprol (BAL), can be given without serious side effects under close medical supervision if care is taken during manufacture to provide enough BAL in the preparation. Otherwise, abdominal colic, severe diarrhea, exfoliative dermatitis, hepatitis, and encephalopathy might occur and require BAL therapy.

VASCULAR INFECTIONS

Bacteremia

TREATMENT OF CHOICE	ALTERNATE
S. aureus See treatment of endocarditis (p. 178)	
Pneumococcus See treatment of pneumococcal pneumonia (p. 153)	
H. influenzae See treatment of *H. influenzae* pneumonia (p. 155)	
Gonococcus Penicillin G, 1,000,000 units intravenously every 6 hours for 10 days	Tetracycline, 1.5 gm orally, then 500 mg 4 times daily for 10 days, or cephalothin, 1.0 gm intravenously every 3 hours for 7 days

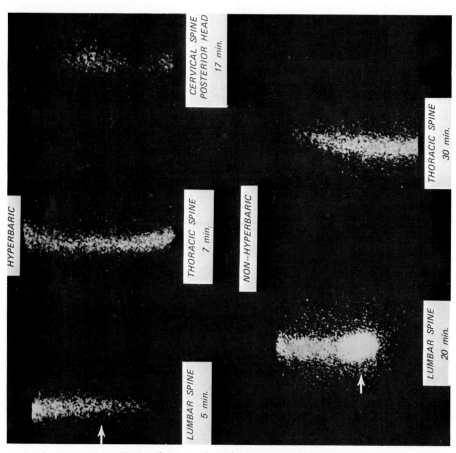

Figure 7–4. *See legend on the opposite page.*

Bacteremia (*Continued*)

TREATMENT OF CHOICE | ALTERNATE

Groups A and B streptococcus, meningococcus, *L. monocytogenes, P. multocida,* and *S. moniliformis*

Penicillin G, 1,000,000 units intravenously every 6 hours for 10 days

Cephalothin, 1.0 gm intravenously every 6 hours for 7–10 days

B. abortus, B. suis, and *B. melitensis*

Tetracycline, 0.5 gm orally 4 times daily for 4 days

Streptomycin, 1.0 gm intramuscularly daily, plus tetracycline, 0.5 gm orally 4 times daily for 10 days

Peptostreptococcus, C. perfringens, and *Bacteroides* other than *B. fragilis*

Penicillin G, 2,000,000 units intravenously every 4 hours

Clindamycin, 300 mg intravenously every 4 hours

E. coli, P. mirabilis

Ampicillin, 2.0 gm intravenously every 3 hours, or kanamycin, 0.5 gm intramuscularly 4 times daily

Gentamicin, 100 mg intravenously every 8 hours

Salmonella typhosa and other salmonellae

Ampicillin, 2.0 gm intravenously every 6 hours for 14 days, or chloramphenicol, 1.0 gm orally every 6 hours until afebrile, then 0.5 gm every 6 hours for 14 days

Trimethoprim, 160 mg, and sulfamethoxazole, 800 mg orally every 12 hours[93]

P. aeruginosa

Carbenicillin, 2.5 gm intravenously every 2 hours, plus gentamicin, 100 mg intravenously every 8 hours

Polymyxin B sulfate, 50 mg in 300 ml 5% dextrose by continuous intravenous drip every 8 hours (total dose 150 mg)

K. pneumoniae

Kanamycin, 0.5 gm intramuscularly every 6 hours, or gentamicin, 100 mg intravenously every 8 hours

Carbenicillin, 2.0 gm intravenously every 2 hours

Figure 7–4. Above: Hyperbaric cisternogram of a patient with coccidioidal meningitis. Scintiphotos are shown from the lumbar injection site (arrow), thoracic spine and upper cervical spine and head after intrathecal injection of dextrose in water and radioisotope with the patient in Trendelenburg position. Note that most of the radioactivity has cleared from the lumbar spine five minutes after injection. Tracer is seen in the head 17 minutes after injection. *Below:* Conventional cisternogram of the same patient with coccidioidal meningitis. The scintiphotos show that when a nonhyperbaric radioisotope is injected with the patient lying flat, 20 minutes after injection there is considerable activity remaining in the lumbar region at the injection site (arrow) and sparse activity above the thoracic level 30 minutes after intrathecal injection. (From Alazraki NP: Use of a hyperbaric solution for administration of intrathecal amphotericin B. N Engl J Med 290:645, 1974.)

Bacteremia (*Continued*)

TREATMENT OF CHOICE	ALTERNATE

E. aerogenes, S. marcescens, indole + *Proteus*

Gentamicin, 100 mg intravenously every 8 hours, plus carbenicillin, 2.0 gm intravenously every 2 hours

Kanamycin, 1.0 gm intramuscularly every 8 hours, plus carbenicillin, 2.0 gm intravenously every 2 hours

Mima polymorpha (*Acinetobacteria*)

Kanamycin, 0.5 gm intramuscularly every 6 hours

Gentamicin, 100 mg intravenously every 8 hours

Plague: *P. pestis*

See treatment of plague pneumonia (p. 155)

Relapsing fever: *Borrelia recurrentis*
Epidemic (louse-borne)

Doxycycline, 100 mg orally for 1 day

Chloramphenicol, 500 mg orally every 6 hours for 10 days for both epidemic and endemic

Endemic (tick-borne)

Tetracycline, 500 mg orally every 6 hours for 10 days

Endocarditis

Viridans, anaerobic, bovis[49] and beta-hemolytic streptococci (except group D), *S. aureus* and *S. epidermidis* (penicillinase-negative), *S. moniliformis, H. aphrophilus*

Penicillin G, 1,000,000 units intravenously every 3 hours for 28 days

Cephalothin, 1.0 gm intravenously every 3 hours, or cefazolin, 1 gm intramuscularly every 8 hours for 28 days

Penicillinase-producing *S. aureus* or *S. epidermidis*

Methicillin or oxacillin, 2.0 gm intravenously every 3 hours for 42 days

Cefazolin, 1 gm intramuscularly every 6 hours, or cephalothin, 2.0 gm intravenously every 4 hours for 42 days

Enterococci

Penicillin G, 2,000,000 units intravenously every 3 hours for 42 days, plus streptomycin, 1.0 gm intramuscularly twice daily for 21 days, then streptomycin, 0.5 gm

Vancomycin, 0.5 gm every 4 hours for 3 days, then every 6 hours for 21 days[35]

Endocarditis (*Continued*)

TREATMENT OF CHOICE   ALTERNATE

intramuscularly twice daily for 21 days; or ampicillin, 2.0 gm intravenously every 3 hours, plus gentamicin, 80 mg intravenously every 8 hours for 42 days

P. aeruginosa

Carbenicillin, 2.5 gm intravenously every 2 hours, plus gentamicin, 100 mg intravenously 4 times daily

Carbenicillin, 2.5 gm intravenously every 2 hours, plus colistin or polymyxin B, 80 mg intravenously every 8 hours

Q fever: *C. burnetii*[65]

Tetracycline, 0.5 gm orally 4 times daily for 30 days, then twice daily for 180 days

Chloramphenicol, 0.5 gm orally 4 times daily for 30 days, then twice daily for 180 days

C. albicans[85]

5-Fluorocytosine, 1.0 gm every 3 hours for 42 days

None

B. abortus, *B. suis*, or *B. melitensis*

See treatment of brucella bacteremia (p. 177)

Parasitemia

Malaria: *Plasmodium vivax*, *P. ovale*, and *P. malariae*

Choloroquine, 600 mg orally for 1 dose; then 300 mg in 6 hours, and then 300 daily for 2 days (total 1.5 base), plus primaquine, 15 mg orally for 14 days.

Amodiaquine dihydrochloride, 600 mg orally then 400 mg daily for 2 days, plus primaquine, 15 mg orally for 14 days

Plasmodium falciparum

Quinine sulfate, 650 mg orally, plus pyrimethamine, 25 gm orally every 12 hours for 3 days, plus sulfadiazine, 500 mg orally every 6 hours for 5 days (Fig. 7–5)

Quinine dihydrochloride, 650 mg in 500 ml saline every 8 hours by slow drip until oral therapy is possible

Hemoflagellates: Trypanosomes, *T. rhodesiense*

Suramin, 200 mg intravenously, then 1 gm intravenously on days 1, 3, 7, 14, and 21

Pentamidine, 250 mg intramuscularly daily for 10 days

Parasitemia (*Continued*)

TREATMENT OF CHOICE	ALTERNATE

T. gambiense
Pentamidine, 250 mg intramuscularly daily for 10 days

Suramin, 200 mg intravenously then 1.0 gm on days 1, 3, 7, 14, and 21

Filariasis *Wuchereria bancrofti*
Diethylcarbamazine, 150 mg orally 4 times daily for 14 days

None

Fungemia

C. albicans
See treatment of endocarditis

Amphotericin B, 40 mg every other day (total 800 mg)

C. neoformans
See treatment of meningitis (p. 171)

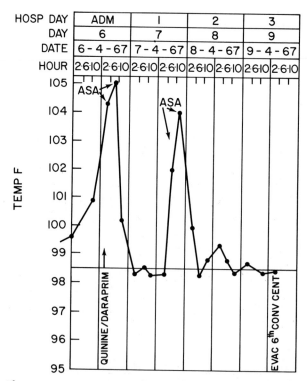

Figure 7–5. The temperature response to therapy of a patient with acute falciparum malaria. Note final paroxysm of fever on second day of therapy. Patients should be forewarned of this paroxysm. (From Blount RE, Teschan PE: Acute falciparum malaria, field experience with quinine/pyrimethamine combined therapy. Ann Intern Med 70(1):144, 1969.)

The successful treatment of bacteremia must not only eliminate bacteria from the blood but also eradicate their source. Inability to clear bacteria from the blood seems to be the primary problem in gram-negative bacterial infections in neutropenic and other immunosuppressed patients who sustain bacteremias from inconsequential foci in the rectum, bowel, nasopharynx, decubiti, or female genitalia. These bacteremias start explosively, often with shock, and require urgent treatment long before the bacteria in the blood can be identified. Since gentamicin and carbenicillin will cover most possibilities, including *P. aeruginosa*, this combination has been recommended for beginning treatment of acute bacteremias.[6] Survival rates with these two drugs in combination are reported to be as good in neutropenic patients as survival after treating with a combination of five drugs.[96] The main objection to the gentamicin-carbenicillin regimen has been its uncertain coverage of associated staphylococcal bacteremia. Since cephalothin or cefazolin would cover staphylococci and also contribute to the treatment of *E. coli*, *K. pneumoniae*, and *P. mirabilis* bacteremias, a triple combination of a cephalosporin, gentamicin, and carbenicillin would be reasonable for starting treatment of bacteremia. After bacteria are isolated in culture, treatment can be adjusted on the basis of sensitivity tests.

In bacteremic patients who are not immunosuppressed or neutropenic, the *focus* is the major problem and must be attacked even more vigorously than the circulating organisms. Some foci can be treated with antibiotics alone, while others can only be eliminated by surgery. Bacteremias arising from kidneys and biliary trees obstructed by stones, or from abscesses, require relief of obstruction and drainage. On the other hand, vegetations in endocarditis, lymphatic and reticuloendothelial foci in typhoid fever or brucellosis, thrombophlebitic foci in staphylococcal and *Bacteroides* septicemia, the pneumonias in pneumococcal and *Klebsiella* bacteremias, the genital or rectal infections in gonococcal septicemia, and the pharyngeal sites feeding meningococci into the blood can all be controlled with antibiotics alone. Septic thrombophlebitis due to *B. fragilis* is probably the most difficult of these to sterilize because of the relative resistance of the organism and its inaccessibility within the long narrow venous clot. In pelvic thrombophlebitis, heparin should be given in conjunction with antibiotics, and ligation of the inferior vena cava may be necessary in some patients.

It is generally assumed in bacterial endocarditis that antibiotics must be given in high enough doses to produce "bactericidal" levels in the vegetation because most of the organisms are beyond the reach of phagocytic cells that would otherwise destroy or remove them. Bactericidal levels generally mean concentrations of the antibiotic that kill all, or nearly all, bacteria in a standard inoculum in the test tube, and the sera of patients under treatment for endocarditis are often examined to see if they can kill the bacteria isolated from the blood. The idea that bactericidal levels are needed for curing endocarditis gained early support from the observation that penicillin plus streptomycin killed the enterococcus and cured enterococcal endocarditis, while each drug alone did neither.[52, 64] Yet no controlled clinical observations have been done to prove that bactericidal levels in the blood are required to cure endocarditis. On the other hand, there are good studies to indicate that duration of treatment may be more important than the daily dose of antibiotic.[20] During the period needed to cure endocarditis the phagocytic cells and antibiotics probably both participate in destroying the infection.[80] The vegetation is slowly invaded from valvular tissues by phagocytic cells while organisms on the vegetation are either inhibited or killed by the antibiotic. It is conceivable, for example, that a bacteriostatic drug could suppress bacteremia long enough to allow an endocardial infection to be overcome by the phagocytic process invading the vegetation from the valve leaflet. While many patients can be cured of endocarditis in two weeks, at least three weeks are required for uniform recovery from endocarditis due to the viridans group of streptococci and six weeks for staphylococci, enterococci, and other resistant organisms. For practical purposes staphylococcal bacteremia should be treated as though endocarditis were present, because the risk of endocarditis approaches 70 per cent in staphylococcal bacteremia.[69]

If antibiotics cannot sterilize the vegetation, the infected valve must be removed surgically and replaced by a prosthesis. Surgery is required mainly for mycotic endocarditis, but certain resistant bacterial infections, such as *Pseudomonas* endocarditis, may also require valvulectomy. Surgery is also indicated for patients with fulminant aortic valvular destruction and decompensation even if the bacteria are very sensitive to antibiotics.[13]

The successful treatment of parasitemia also requires elimination of tissue foci. In all forms of malaria except falciparum, for example, primaquine must be used to eliminate infection of the hepatic parenchymal cells. Chloroquine cures only the erythrocytic phase, and the patient will suffer a relapse if the secondary tissue schizont in the liver is not destroyed by primaquine. *P. falciparum* presents a special problem, however, because it develops chloroquine resistance.[79] Patients who acquire falciparum malaria in Asia or South America should be treated with quinine, pyrimethamine, and sulfadiazine. In Africa, on the other hand, *P. falciparum* remains sensitive to chloroquine. In acute trypanosomiasis the trypanosomes are present in the blood, lymph nodes, liver, and spleen, and suramin or pentamidine can destroy organisms in all sites. Similarly in bancroftian filariasis, diethylcarbamazine kills both the adult female worms in the lymphatics or connective tissues and the microfilariae which are set free into the circulation.[60]

DERMAL INFECTIONS

Pyogenic Infections

TREATMENT OF CHOICE	ALTERNATE

Furunculosis: S. *aureus* (penicillinase-negative)

Penicillin V, 1.0 gm orally 4 times daily	Cephalexin, 0.5 gm, plus probenecid, 0.5 gm orally 4 times daily

S. *aureus* (penicillinase-positive)

Dicloxacillin, 0.5 gm orally 4 times daily	Cephalexin, 0.5 gm, plus probenecid, 0.5 gm orally 4 times daily, or erythromycin, 0.5 gm orally 4 times daily

Pyoderma and impetigo: group A streptococcus

Benzathine penicillin, 1,200,000 units intramuscularly for 1 day, or penicillin V, 500 mg orally 4 times daily for 10 days	Erythromycin or cephalexin, 250 mg orally 4 times daily for 10 days

Streptococcal cellulitis and erysipelas: group A streptococcus

Procaine penicillin, 600,000 units intramuscularly twice daily until afebrile, then penicillin V, 500 mg orally 4 times daily for 10 days	Cefazolin, 1.0 gm intramuscularly twice daily until afebrile, then cephalexin, 500 mg orally 4 times daily for 10 days

Pseudomonas cellulitis: *P. aeruginosa*

Gentamicin, 80 mg intramuscularly 3 times daily	Colistin, 80 mg intramuscularly 3 times daily, or carbenicillin, 1.0 gm intramuscularly 4 times daily

Ecthyma gangrenosum: *P. aeruginosa*

Carbenicillin, 2.0 gm intravenously every 2 hours, plus gentamicin, 80 mg intravenously 3 times daily	Carbenicillin, 2.0 gm intravenously every 2 hours

Skin Infections Acquired from Animals

Bites: *P. multocida*

Penicillin V, 500 mg orally 4 times daily	Cefalexin, 500 mg orally 4 times daily

Tularemia: *F. tularensis*

See treatment of tularemic pneumonia (p. 156)

Skin Infections Acquired from Animals (*Continued*)

TREATMENT OF CHOICE   ALTERNATE

Bubonic plague: *P. pestis*
See treatment of plague pneumonia (p. 155)

Rat-bite fever: *Spirillum minus*
 Procaine penicillin, 600,000 units intramuscularly twice daily for 1 day Tetracycline, 500 mg orally every 6 hours for 7 days

Erysipeloid: *Erysipelothrix insidiosa*
 Benzathine penicillin, 1,200,000 units intramuscularly for 1 day Erythromycin, 250 mg orally 4 times daily for 7 days

Anthrax: *B. anthracis*[40]
 Penicillin V, 500 mg orally 4 times daily for 7 days, or aqueous procaine penicillin, 600,000 units intramuscularly twice daily Tetracycline, 500 mg orally 4 times daily

Typhus
Epidemic: *Rickettsia prowazekii*[82]
 Doxycycline, 200 mg orally for 1 day Chloramphenicol, 3.5 gm orally or intravenously, then 1.0 gm every 8 hours until afebrile 48 hours and for at least 12 days

Endemic: *Rickettsia mooseri*
 Chloramphenicol as in epidemic typhus

Rocky Mountain spotted fever: *Rickettsia rickettsii*
 Doxycycline, 200 mg orally daily until afebrile, then 100 mg daily for total course of 12 days Chloramphenicol as in typhus

Scrub typhus: *Rickettsia tsutsugamushi*
 Chloramphenicol as in typhus

Dermal Fungus Infections

Blastomycosis: *B. dermatitidis*
See treatment of pulmonary blastomycosis (p. 156)

Sporotrichosis: *Sporothrix schenckii*
 Saturated potassium iodide orally, 10 drops 3 times daily after meals increased to tolerance; continue for 1 month after lesions disappear Amphotericin B, 40 mg intravenously every other day (total 1.6 gm)

Dermal Fungus Infections (*Continued*)

Chromoblastomycosis

5-Fluorocytosine, 1.0 gm orally every 4 hours, plus 1% sol topically[72] or amphotericin B (0.5% in 2% procaine sol) injected into lesions once weekly for 12 weeks[24]

Potassium iodide as in sporotrichosis plus calciferol, 600,000 units intramuscularly once weekly

Moniliasis (intertrigo and paronychia): *C. albicans*

Mycostatin ointment or powder (100,000 units per gram) topically twice daily or crystal violet (1% sol) topically

Miconazole nitrate ointment (2%) or amphotericin B lotion (2%) applied to lesions twice daily

Chronic mucocutaneous moniliasis

Amphotericin B, 30 mg intravenously every other day (total 450–900 mg)

5-Fluorocytosine, 2.0 gm orally every 6 hours

Mycobacterial, Venereal, and Nonvenereal Treponemal Infections

Sporotrichoid mycobacterial infection: *M. marinum* and *M. kansasii*

Rifampin, 600 mg, and ethambutol, 1.0 gm orally daily[105]

Streptomycin, 0.5 gm intramuscularly, plus rifampin, 600 mg orally daily

M. intracellulare

Isoniazid, 300 mg, rifampin, 600 mg, and ethambutol, 1.0 gm orally daily

Leprosy[98]

Dapsone, 100 mg orally daily

Clofazimine, 100 mg orally daily

Syphilis
Yaws
Pinta
Bejel
} See treatment of oropharyngeal infections (p. 151)

Chancroid: *Hemophilus ducreyi*

Sulfadiazine, 1.0 gm orally 4 times daily for 5–7 days

Tetracycline, 0.5 gm 4 times daily for 10 days

Parasitic Infestations

Filariasis: *Onchocerca volvulus*

Suramin, 200 mg intravenously,   None

Parasitic Infestations (*Continued*)

<table>
<tr><td>TREATMENT OF CHOICE</td><td>ALTERNATE</td></tr>
</table>

then 1.0 gm intravenously weekly
for 5 weeks, plus diethylcarbamazine, 25 mg orally daily for
3 days, 50 mg daily for 5 days, 100
mg daily for 3 days, and then 150
mg daily for 12 days

Loa Loa
    Diethylcarbamazine, 200 mg orally   None
    3 times daily for 14–21 days

Dracunculus medinensis
    Niridazole, 500 mg orally 3   None
    times daily with meals for 10
    days[73]

Cutaneous larva migrans (creeping eruption): *Ancylostoma brasiliensis* and
A. caninum
    Thiabendazole, 1.5 gm orally twice   None
    daily for 3 days after meals

Anaerobic Cellulitis

Anaerobic streptococci: *C. perfringens*
    Penicillin G, 2,000,000 units intra-   Clindamycin, 600 mg intrave-
    venously every 6 hours   nously every 8 hours

B. fragilis
    Clindamycin, 600 mg intrave-   Chloramphenicol, 1.0 gm orally or
    nously every 8 hours   intravenously every 6 hours

Dermatophytosis

Microsporum and *Trichophyton* spp.
    Topical tolnaftate (1%) or micon-   Griseofulvin, 250 mg orally 4
    azole nitrate (2%)   times daily

Accessibility of skin lesions allows topical use of tolnaftate, miconazole, bacitracin, gentamicin, and other antimicrobial drugs for some mild superficial infections, such as mild forms of dermatophytosis and impetigo, but systemic drugs are usually indicated. Most bacterial infections can be treated with one of the penicillins. Not only staphylococcal, group A streptococcal, and clostridial infections respond to benzylpenicillin, but anthrax, erysipeloid, and *P. multocida* infections and syphilis are cured by it. The main exceptions are leprosy and other mycobacterial infections. Dapsone is the standard drug for leprosy, but treatment of anonymous mycobacterial infections varies with individual drug sensitivity. Usually combinations of rifampin with streptomycin or ethambutol are used in sporotrichoid and other forms of *M. kansasii* or *M. marinum* infections. Application of heat is also important because most strains of *M. marinum* cannot survive at temperatures above 32 to 33° C, and some cases have been cured by hot applications without drugs. Topical heat is also valuable for classical sporotrichosis due to *S. schenckii* and is reported to have cured sporotrichosis in patients who did not receive or could not tolerate iodides or amphotericin B.

As in infections elsewhere, debridement and abscess drainage are essential for the cure of certain skin infections. Debridement is probably more important than drugs for anaerobic skin infections. This is especially the case in diabetic infections of the feet and legs. Since anaerobic bacteria are killed at the oxidation-reduction potential (eH) of normal body fluids, it is doubtful if antibiotics can add much to the antibacterial properties of plasma or lymph except by diffusing into the dying ischemic tissues and arresting the spread of anaerobes at the periphery of early infections. In the mouth, liver, lung, or brain, where there is an excellent blood supply, anaerobic cellulitis can be arrested in this fashion and the small areas of necrosis reabsorbed. In the diabetic foot, on the other hand, the extremely poor vascular supply cannot deliver the drug, and the results even with high doses are poor even after extensive debridement or amputation. Hyperbaric oxygen can sometimes arrest nonclostridial anaerobic cellulitis in diabetics when antibiotics fail and extensive debridement is not feasible.

Treatment of parasitic infestations of the skin continues to improve in effectiveness as better drugs become available, but some of these are toxic. Niridazole produces headache, dizziness, fever, nausea, and abdominal pain in some patients and changes the color of the urine to a deep brown-black color. Convulsions and tremors are more serious reactions that are seen occasionally. Suramin may be nephrotoxic and must be used with great caution in patients with renal disease. It may also cause conjunctivitis, stomatitis, peripheral neuritis, and agranulocytosis. Diethylcarbamazine is usually well-tolerated, but severe allergic reactions occur due to the rapid massive destruction of microfilaria in onchocerciasis, and both microfilaria and adult worms in loiasis (see Chapter 6). These allergic reactions can be controlled by steroids and antihistamines. Worm removal is an important adjunct to treatment in some cases of skin filariasis. In onchocerciasis the load of adult worms can be substantially reduced by simply excising nodules, and "guinea worms" can be readily removed after a course of niridazole for *Dracunculus medinensis*.

Perhaps the most remarkable new development in treatment is the discovery that one dose of doxycycline will cure epidemic typhus. The drug has not been used enough in scrub typhus or endemic typhus to evaluate its effectiveness, and chloramphenicol is recommended instead. The lipid solubility of doxycycline could explain its remarkable effectiveness in epidemic typhus, since intracellular penetration of endothelial cells infected with rickettsiae would be facilitated by lipid solubility.

OCULAR INFECTIONS

Blepharoconjunctivitis

TREATMENT OF CHOICE | ALTERNATE

S. aureus, pneumococcus, group A streptococcus, *H. influenzae, P. aeruginosa, H. aegyptus*

Topical gentamicin, 0.3% sol, 2 drops every hour for 24 days, then 2 drops every 3 hours

Gentamicin ointment, 0.3% in white petrolatum 3 times daily and at bedtime

Gonococcal

Topical penicillin G, 0.6% sol, 2 drops every hour until acute inflammation subsides; then 2 drops every 3 hours plus 600,000 units procaine penicillin daily

Gentamicin, 0.3% sol as for *S. aureus*, plus tetracycline HCl, 1.5 gm orally

Chlamydial (TRIC Agents) Keratoconjunctivitis

Trachoma

Chlortetracycline ointment, 1.0% in white petrolatum 4 times daily for 60 days, plus sulfisoxazole, 1.0 gm every 6 hours orally

Erythromycin ointment, 0.5% in mineral oil and white petrolatum 4 times daily for 60 days, plus sulfisoxazole, 1.0 gm orally every 6 hours

Inclusion conjunctivitis

Topical chlortetracycline, 1% sol every 2 hours for 5 days then 4 times daily for 14 days, plus tetracycline HCl, 500 mg orally for 21 days or doxycycline 200 mg, then 100 mg orally daily for 21 days

Topical erythromycin lactobionate, 0.5% sol every 2 hours for 5 days, then 4 times daily for 14 days, plus erythromycin, 500 mg orally 4 times daily for 21 days

Viral Keratoconjunctivitis

Herpes simplex

5-Iodo-2-deoxyuridine, 0.1% sol in distilled H_2O, 1 drop in eye every hour in daytime and every 2 hours at night until fluorescein staining disappears; then 1 drop every 2

5-Iodo-2-deoxyuridine, 0.5% in petroleum base ointment instilled into conjunctival sac every 4 hours until 5 days after complete healing

Viral Keratoconjunctivitis (Continued)

TREATMENT OF CHOICE   ALTERNATE

hours in daytime and every 4 hours at night for 5 days after complete healing

Herpes zoster
Dexamethasone phosphate solution, 0.1%, 1 drop hourly while awake for 14 days, then tapered over next 14 days

None

Bacterial Keratoconjunctivitis

S. aureus, group A streptococcus, pneumococcus, *P. aeruginosa*
Gentamicin as for conjunctivitis plus topical dexamethasone phosphate sol

Subconjunctival gentamicin, 20 mg/ml daily

Gonococcal
Same as conjunctivitis plus topical dexamethasone phosphate sol

Mycotic Keratoconjunctivitis

Aspergillus fumigatus, *Candida* sp., *Fusarium* sp., *Fusidium* sp., *Gibberella* sp., *Neurospora* sp., *Penicillium* sp., *Allescheria boydii*, *Curvalaria* sp.
Amphotericin B, 0.1% sol in 0.9% NaCl sol, 1 drop topically to eye every hour until improvement; then at increasing intervals; continue for 2 weeks after healing

Nystatin, 2000 units/ml 0.9% saline sol, topically to eye as described for amphotericin B

Endophthalmitis

S. epidermidis, *S. aureus*, nonhemolytic streptococci, pneumococcus, *E. coli*
Chloramphenicol, 1.0 gm orally every 6 hours, plus chloramphenicol succinate, 1.0 gm intravenously every 6 hours, plus gentamicin, 60 mg by subtenon injection for 1 dose

Ampicillin, 2.5 gm every 3 hours intravenously (or methicillin, 2.5 gm every 3 hours intravenously for penicillinase-producing staphylococci), plus 1 subtenon injection of gentamicin, 60 mg

P. aeruginosa
Carbenicillin, 2.5 gm intravenously every 2 hours, plus gentamicin, 60 mg by subtenon injection for 1 dose

Carbenicillin, 2.5 gm intravenously, plus 0.4 mg gentamicin, plus 0.36 mg dexamethasone in 0.1 ml volume by one direct intravitreous injection

Uveitis

Toxoplasma gondii
  See treatment of toxoplasmosis of lung (p. 153)
T. pallidum
  See treatment of oral syphilis (p. 151)
C. neoformans
  5-Fluorocytosine as in cryptococcal
  meningitis

Although gentamicin would not be the drug of choice for treating systemic infections caused by the bacteria that produce conjunctivitis, it is highly effective against all of them in a 0.3% solution (3000 μg/ml) because this concentration is 100 times that needed to inhibit even the more resistant bacteria that infect the eye.[63] While penicillin is listed as the drug of choice for gonococcal ophthalmitis by most authorities, topical gentamicin would probably be effective for this infection as well because the gonococcus is inhibited by 1.6 μg/ml or less of gentamicin.[63] Other topical antibiotics can be used as well, but none combine the broad spectrum and efficacy of gentamicin. The major exception to gentamicin therapy is in chlamydial infection for which either topical chlortetracycline or erythromycin is remarkably effective.

The accessibility of the cornea to topical therapy allows the successful use of other drugs that cannot be used systemically. The most important of these is idoxuridine which can cure *Herpes simplex* keratitis. It is not indicated in *Herpes zoster* infection, however, and steroids should be used instead. Both topical and systemic steroid therapy is of value in ophthalmic zoster to prevent scarring and postherpetic neuralgia of the optic nerve. Steroids should never be used alone in simplex keratitis.

Topical therapy is much less effective in fungal keratitis and endophthalmitis.[58] Isolation of the fungus and sensitivity testing to amphotericin, mycostatin, 5-fluorocytosine, and miconazole[100] are warranted in order to choose the right drug. Special topical preparations would have to be made up with the latter two, but they might be valuable for topical and systemic therapy in this otherwise discouraging infection. Frequently a thin conjunctival flap is effective in treating mycotic ulcers when drugs fail.[58]

Chloramphenicol is listed as the drug of choice for endophthalmitis because it penetrates better after systemic therapy than others. It is inactive, however, against *P. aeruginosa*, and the only hope for treating this organism would be carbenicillin systemically and gentamicin by subtenon or intravitreous injection. Local and systemic corticosteroids are important accessory treatment for endophthalmitis and keratitis when antimicrobial drugs are known to be effective in controlling the infection. Steroids minimize scarring and reduce damage from inflammation in the eye.[4]

MUSCULOSKELETAL INFECTIONS

Septic Arthritis or Tenosynovitis

Treatment of Choice	Alternate

Pneumococcus, gonococcus, group A streptococcus, *S. aureus* (penicillinase-negative), meningococcus, *S. moniliformis*

Penicillin G, 1,000,000 units intravenously every 6 hours

Cephalothin, 1.0 gm intravenously every 3 hours

B. abortus, B. suis, B. melitensis

Tetracycline, 0.5 gm orally 4 times daily

Tetracycline, 0.5 gm orally 4 times daily, plus streptomycin, 1.0 gm intramuscularly daily

B. fragilis

Clindamicin, 600 mg intravenously every 6 hours

Chloramphenicol, 2.0 gm orally every 8 hours

M. tuberculosis

Isoniazid, 300 mg orally daily

Rifampin, 600 mg orally daily

M. kansasii

See treatment of sporotrichoid mycobacterial infections (p. 185)

M. intracellulare

Isoniazid, 300 mg, plus ethambutol, 1.0 gm, plus rifampin, 600 mg orally daily

None

***Salmonella* spp.**

Chloramphenicol, 0.5 gm orally every 3 hours

Ampicillin, 2.0 gm intravenously every 6 hours

E. coli, P. mirabilis

Ampicillin, 2.0 gm intravenously every 3 hours, or kanamycin, 0.5 gm intramuscularly 4 times daily

Gentamicin, 100 mg intravenously every 8 hours

P. aeruginosa

Gentamicin, 80 mg intravenously every 8 hours, plus carbenicillin, 2.0 gm intravenously every 2 hours

Gentamicin or polymyxin B, 5.0 mg intra-articularly, plus hydrocortisone, 25 mg every other day for 4 days

S. schenckii

Amphotericin B, 40–60 mg intravenously every other day[59]

None

Acute Hematogenous Osteomyelitis

TREATMENT OF CHOICE   ALTERNATE

S. *aureus* (penicillinase-negative)

Penicillin G, 1,000,000 units intra- Cephalothin, 1.0 gm intravenously
venously every 8 hours for 28 days; every 8 hours for 28 days; then
then penicillin V, 1.0 gm orally 4 cephalexin, 1.0 gm orally 4 times
times daily for 28 days   daily, plus probenecid, 0.5 gm 4
                                    times daily for 28 days[55, 62]

S. *aureus* (penicillinase-positive)

Methicillin or oxacillin, 2.0 gm in- Cephalothin and cephalexin as for
travenously every 4 hours for 28 penicillinase-negative S. *aureus*
days, then dicloxacillin, 0.5 gm
orally every 6 hours for 21 days

P. *aeruginosa*[45, 70]

Carbenicillin, 2.5 gm intravenously Colistin or polymyxin B, 80 mg
every 2 hours, plus gentamicin, 80 intramuscularly every 8 hours
mg intravenously every 8 hours

Salmonella spp.

Ampicillin, 1.0 gm intravenously Trimethoprim, 160 mg, and sulfa-
every 4 hours, or chloramphenicol, methoxazole, 800 mg orally every
1.0 gm orally every 6 hours 12 hours

M. *tuberculosis*

Isoniazid, 300 mg orally daily Rifampin, 600 mg orally daily

B. *abortus*, B. *suis*, and B. *melitensis*
See treatment of arthritis (p. 191)

Chronic Osteomyelitis

S. *aureus* (penicillinase-negative)

Penicillin V, 1.0 gm, plus proben- Cephalexin, 1.0 gm 4 times daily,
ecid, 0.5 gm orally 4 times daily, or trimethoprim, 160 mg, plus sulfa-
or tetracycline, 0.5 gm orally 4 methoxazole, 800 mg orally every
times daily   12 hours

S. *aureus* (penicillinase-positive)

Dicloxacillin or oxacillin, 0.5 gm, Same as for penicillinase-negative
plus probenecid, 0.5 gm orally S. *aureus*
4 times daily

A. *israelii*

See treatment of actinomycosis of the jaw (p. 150)

Chronic Osteomyelitis (Continued)

TREATMENT OF CHOICE   ALTERNATE

Mycetoma ("madura foot"): *Streptomyces madurae* and *Nocardia brasiliensis*

Trisulfapyrimidines, 1.0 gm orally   None
every 4 hours

M. tuberculosis

See treatment of acute tuberculosis of the bone (p. 192)

B. dermatitidis, C. immitis, and *C. neoformans*

Same as pulmonary infections   Local irrigation into sinuses of
amphotericin B, 0.5% sol with
0.1% hydrocortisone

Myositis

Gas gangrene: *C. perfringens, C. novyi*

Penicillin G, 1.0 gm intravenously   Cephalothin, 1.0 gm intravenously
every 2 hours   every 2 hours

Hematogenous osteomyelitis and septic arthritis respond to the same treatment as the underlying bacteremia because antibiotic penetration gives levels in joints and bones that are more or less the same as in the blood. Treatment must be started soon enough in staphylococcal osteomyelitis to prevent irreversible changes.[46] Otherwise, there is a danger of large avascular sequestra that harbor bacteria and insulate them against antibiotics in the blood.[54] Because staphylococcal septicemia itself is often alarming and fulminating, patients with hematogenous osteomyelitis are usually given treatment with large doses of antibiotics so that the septicemia as well as the osteomyelitis is soon arrested. At least 70 per cent of acute staphylococcal osteomyelitis is cured,[53] and often without surgical intervention. In some patients, however, subperiosteal abscesses and intramedullary pus must be drained during drug therapy. The length of treatment is as important as an early start; acute osteomyelitis is more likely to progress to a chronic infection in patients given a short course of treatment.[101] Most authorities recommend at least one month of parenteral treatment.

The picture of osteomyelitis with gram-negative bacteria is entirely different than that presented by the *Staphylococcus*. Gram-negative organisms do not present the life-threatening generalized illness with rapid destruction of growing long bones in children that is characteristic of staphylococcal osteomyelitis. Instead, gram-negative bacilli usually produce low-grade spinal osteomyelitis in adults following urinary infection or heroin injection, and often without fever or leukocytosis.[39, 70, 71] The prognosis is excellent and many patients recover with bed rest alone. Staphylococci may also produce spinal osteomyelitis in adults, while gram-negative organisms may occasionally infect long bones if these are already the seat of another disease such as sickle cell disease, myeloma, compound fracture, Gaucher's disease, or leukemia. In other situations the pathogenic significance of gram-negative bacteria in long bones is sometimes questionable because these organisms may simply be superficial contaminants that mask underlying staphylococci by overgrowth in culture.

Chronic staphylococcal osteomyelitis almost always requires a combination of surgery and antibiotics. Some authorities advocate radical excision of sinus tracts, abscess walls, dead bone, and all scar tissue, with primary closure of the surgical wound under antibiotic coverage.[21] Others obtain good results by avoiding extensive surgical procedures and confining themselves to drainage of abscesses, removal of retained sequestra, and meticulous attention to antibiotic levels.[10] Apparent cure has been reported after prolonged treatment with doses of oral penicillins that give one-hour serum levels greater than 25 μg/ml and three-hour readings of 5 μg/ml. These levels can be achieved if probenecid is used and if care is taken to give the antibiotic after a fast for three hours (i.e., one hour before the next meal). When treatment is continued for at least six months or until all signs of disease are gone, most patients seem to be cured by such antibiotic treatment if abscesses are drained and sequestra removed.[10] In patients who cannot be cured by a penicillin, oral treatment is continued indefinitely to suppress drainage and prevent pain. In some patients tetracycline is more effective than the penicillins, possibly because of its unique localization in bone.

Aside from the *Staphylococcus* the major causes of chronic bone infection are actinomycosis, tuberculosis, fungi, and the organisms that cause mycetoma. Patients with actinomycosis and tuberculosis consistently recover after drug treatment, but the other infections are variable in their response. Among the fungi, blastomycosis responds better than coccidioidomycosis to amphotericin B. In fact, there is serious question as to whether systemic amphotericin acccomplishes anything for patients with coccidioidomycosis of bone. Local infusion of amphotericin into bone sinuses may be of slight value but, in general, the drug is disappointing. The same is true for amphotericin therapy of mycetoma caused by *Aspergillus, Cephalosporium, Phialophora,* and *Allescheria boydii,* and many cases require amputation. Better results are obtained with sulfonamides in mycetomas caused by *Streptomyces* and *Nocardia.*

Penicillin is given as standard therapy in gas gangrene of muscle because clostridia are very sensitive to the antibiotic *in vitro.* The value of clostridial antiserum is questionable. The only proved treatment is amputation of the tissues or limb. Hyperbaric oxygen may be of value in some cases.

DRUG PROPHYLAXIS OF INFECTIONS

Bacterial

PROPHYLAXIS OF CHOICE	ALTERNATE

Group A streptococcus: sore throat and rheumatic fever[87]

Benzathine penicillin, 1,200,000 units intramuscularly monthly, or penicillin V, 250 mg orally twice daily

Sulfadiazine, 1.0 gm daily, or erythromycin, 500 mg orally twice daily

Pneumococcal infection in agammaglobulinemia

Same as for group A streptococcus

Meningococcal infections

Rifampin, 600 mg orally daily for 4 days[27]

Minocycline, 100 mg every 12 hours for 5 days[29]

Tuberculosis[33]

Isoniazid, 300 mg orally daily for 1 year

None

Gonococcal ophthalmia

1% silver nitrate

None

Cholera

Tetracycline, 250 mg orally twice daily

None

Chronic bronchopulmonary infections (acute exacerbations)

Ampicillin, 500 mg 3 times daily, or tetracycline, 500 mg 3 times daily orally for 10 days

Trimethoprim, 160 mg, and sulfamethoxazole, 800 mg orally every 12 hours for 10 days

Indwelling catheters

Continuous bladder rinse with neomycin, 40 mg, and polymyxin B, 20 mg per liter of isotonic saline

1/4% acetic acid bladder rinse

Pyelonephritis of pregnancy

See treatment of bladder bacilluria (p. 164)

Recurrent cystitis

Nitrofurantoin, 50 mg, or buffered penicillin G, 500 mg orally immediately after sexual intercourse

Trimethoprim, 40 mg, and sulfamethoxazole, 200 mg orally daily

Bacterial (*Continued*)

PROPHYLAXIS OF CHOICE	ALTERNATE

Recurrent pyelonephritis in chronic prostatitis[94]
    Ampicillin, 250 mg orally twice daily   Oxytetracycline, 250 mg orally twice daily

Urinary infection after prostatectomy
    Kanamycin, 0.5 gm intramuscularly daily for 2 days   Gentamicin, 80 mg intramuscularly daily for 2 days

Recurrent otitis media in children
    Sulfisoxazole, 0.5–1.0 gm orally twice daily[83]   Ampicillin, 250 mg orally twice daily

Penetrating wounds and compound fractures
    Procaine penicillin, 800,000 units intramuscularly, then dicloxacillin, 250 mg orally 4 times daily   Cefazolin, 0.5 gm intramuscularly, then cephalexin, 500 mg orally twice daily

Viral

Influenza A_2
    Amantadine hydrochloride, 100 mg orally every 12 hours for 8 days   None

Smallpox[9]
    Methisazone, 3.0 gm orally every 12 hours for 1 day within 7 days of exposure   None

Parasitic

Malaria

P. vivax
    Chloroquine, 300 mg, plus primaquine, 45 mg once weekly orally 2 weeks before and 8 weeks after exposure   Amodiaquine dihydrochloride, 520 mg once weekly orally 2 weeks before and 8 weeks after exposure

P. falciparum
    Dapsone, 25 mg daily, plus chloroquine, 300 mg orally once weekly   Pyrimethamine, 25 mg plus chloroquine 300 mg orally once weekly

Trypanosomiasis

T. gambiense
    Pentamidine isethionate, 250 mg intramuscularly every 6 months   None

Parasitic (Continued)

PROPHYLAXIS OF CHOICE   ALTERNATE

Filariasis

Bancroftian filariasis
  Diethylcarbamazine, 400 mg orally   None
  1 day per month

Although most of these chemoprophylactic regimens are well established, they have their limitations and questionable aspects. Rheumatic fever prophylaxis is probably the most widely practiced of these, and its effectiveness in preventing clinical attacks of rheumatic fever is unquestioned. Yet serious doubts have been raised about its ability to prevent rheumatic valvular disease. It is logical to assume that prevention of the acute symptoms of rheumatic fever is associated with prevention of valvulitis, but the validity of this assumption has not been proved in controlled studies.

A different problem confronts meningococcal prophylaxis. Whereas prophylaxis of streptococcal infection has never been compromised by the development of penicillin resistance on the part of group A streptococci, meningococcal prophylaxis has suffered a serious setback through the development of sulfonamide resistance. Until meningococci became highly resistant to sulfonamides, these compounds were remarkably effective in preventing clinical cases of infection. During World War II a dose of 1 gm of sulfadiazine per day over a period of months virtually eliminated meningococcal meningitis in recruits. Resistance has not developed to penicillin among meningococci, but it has no prophylactic value despite its success in *treating* meningococcal infections because it does not eliminate the meningococcus from the nasopharynx. This paradox might be explained by the failure of penicillin to enter the saliva in sufficient concentration. Only rifampin and minocycline can reduce nasopharyngeal carriage of meningococci and be used for prophylaxis, but the risk of resistance to them still exists. Rifampin-resistant meningococci may develop in over 60 per cent of carriers after mass prophylaxis, but resistance to minocycline has not been encountered.[44]

Acquired resistance has also become an important problem in the prophylaxis of at least one nonbacterial infection. Resistance of falciparum malaria to chloroquine in Southeast Asia and South America has created a serious problem for travelers who might be exposed to this dreadful infection. Fortunately, dapsone is relatively reliable for preventing clinical disease from chloroquine-resistant falciparum infections.[22]

An important new area of drug prophylaxis is developing in the field of virus infections. Amantadine is reported to exert its effect by preventing penetration of influenza A_2 virus into the cell, without hindering its adsorption to cell receptors. Its prophylactic value in man appears limited to infections by A_2 viruses. The compound has antiviral activity *in vitro* against *respiratory syncytial virus* and *parainfluenza* viruses, but these viruses are not sensitive enough to be affected by the concentrations of amantadine that appear in nasal and respiratory secretions when the drug is given in acceptable nontoxic doses.[91]

Methisazone, the other effective antiviral agent, has been successful in the prevention of smallpox. Although it is no substitute for vaccination, it can lower the attack rate in epidemics of nonvaccinated populations by 95 per cent. Eventually, smallpox vaccination may eliminate the prophylactic need for this drug, but it may still be needed for treating the complications of vaccination. Promising results have been reported in the treatment of vaccinia gangrenosa and eczema vaccinatum.

A number of other programs of chemoprophylaxis are advocated and widely practiced, but these are either controversial or not well established. The use of penicillin for preventing bacterial endocarditis after dental manipulation, for example, is recommended by the American Heart Association. This recommendation is made in spite of the fact that no controlled studies have proved its value in patients, that endocarditis has occurred despite the "umbrella" of prophylaxis during tooth extraction, and that experimental studies cast doubt on the value of current recommendations for penicillin prophylaxis in the prevention of the viridans type of streptococcal endocarditis.[31]

Even more controversy has centered about the prophylactic use of antibiotics in surgery. In the two most important areas, cardiac and abdominal surgery, careful and extensive double-blind studies have shown that prophylactic administration of potent antimicrobial drugs in high dosage has not prevented postoperative infections.[23, 56]

REFERENCES

1. Abernathy RS: Antibiotic therapy of lung abscess: effectiveness of penicillin. Dis Chest 53:592–598, 1968.
2. Abernathy RS: Treatment of systemic mycoses. Medicine (Baltimore) 52:385–394, 1973.
3. Alazraki NP, Fierer J, Halpern SE, et al: Use of a hyperbaric solution for administration of intrathecal amphotericin B. N Engl J Med 290:641–646, 1974.
4. Aronson SB, Elliott JH: Ocular Inflammation. St. Louis, The C.V. Mosby Co., 1972.
5. Aserkoff B, Bennett JV: Effect of antibiotic therapy in acute salmonellosis on the fecal excretion of salmonellae. N Engl J Med 281:636–640, 1969.
6. Atkinson K, Kay HE, McElwain TJ: Septicaemia in the neutropenic patient. Br Med J 3:244–247, 1974.
7. Bach MC, Sabath LD, Finland M: Susceptibility of Nocardia asteroides to 45 antimicrobial agents in vitro. Antimicrob Agents Chemother 3:1–8, 1973.
8. Bailey RR, Roberts AP, Gower PE, et al: Prevention of urinary-tract infection with low-dose nitrofurantoin. Lancet 2:1112–1114, 1971.
9. Bauer DJ, St. Vincent L, Kempe CH, et al: Prophylactic treatment of smallpox contacts with N-methylisatin beta-thiosemicarbazone (compound 33T57, Marboran). Lancet 2:494–496, 1963.
10. Bell SM: Oral penicillins in the treatment of chronic staphylococcal osteomyelitis. Lancet 2:295–297, 1968.
11. Bell WJ, Nassif S: Comparison of pyrantel pamoate and piperazine phosphate in the treatment of ascariasis. Am J Trop Med Hyg 20:584–588, 1971.
12. Blake JC: Erythromycin in diphtheria. Lancet 2:1023, 1954.
13. Braniff BA, Shumway NE, Harrison DC: Valve replacement in active bacterial endocarditis. N Engl J Med 276:1464–1467, 1967.

14. Braude AI: Current concepts of pyelonephritis. Medicine (Baltimore) 52:257–264, 1973.

15. Brewin A, Arango L, Hadley WK, et al: High-dose penicillin therapy and pneumococcal pneumonia. JAMA 230:409–413, 1974.

16. Brumfitt W, Pursell R: Double-blind trial to compare ampicillin, cephalexin, co-trimoxazole, and trimethoprim in treatment of urinary infection. Br Med J 2:673–676, 1972.

17. Carroll BR, Nicol CS: Trimethoprim-sulphamethoxazole in the treatment of non-gonococcal urethritis and gonorrhoea. Br J Vener Dis 46:31–33, 1970.

18. Carter, RF: Sensitivity to amphotericin B of the Naegleria sp. isolated from a case of primary amoebic meningoencephalitis. J Clin Pathol 22:470–474, 1969.

19. Cash RA, Northrup RS, Mizanur Rahman ASM: Trimethoprim and sulfamethoxazole in clinical cholera: comparison with tetracycline. J Infect Dis 128:Suppl:749–753, 1973.

20. Cates JE, Christie RV: Subacute bacterial endocarditis; review of 442 patients treated in 14 centres appointed by Penicillin Trials Committee of Medical Research Council. Q J Med 20:93–130, 1951.

21. Clawson DK, Stevenson JK: Treatment of chronic osteomyelitis. Surg Gynecol Obstet 120:59–69, 1965.

22. Clyde DF, Rebert CC, McCarthy VC, et al: Prophylaxis of malaria in man using the sulfones DFD and DDS alone and with chloroquine. Milit Med 136:836–841, 1971.

23. Conte JE Jr, Cohen SN, Roe BB, et al: Antibiotic prophylaxis and cardiac surgery. A prospective double-blind comparison of single-dose versus multiple-dose regimens. Ann Intern Med 76:943–949, 1972.

24. Costello MJ, deFeo CP Jr, Littman ML: Chromoblastomycosis treated with local infiltration of amphotericin B solution. Arch Dermatol 79:98–107, 1959.

25. Davies AH, McFadzean JA, Squires S: Treatment of Vincent's stomatitis with met-ronidazole. Br Med J 1:1149–1150, 1964.

26. Dawborn JK, Castaldi PA, Kilgour A, et al: Prolonged use of trimethoprim-sulphonamide in urinary infection. Med J Aust 1:Suppl:52–57, 1973.

27. Deal WB, Sanders E: Efficacy of rifampin in treatment of meningococcal carriers. N Engl J Med 281:641–645, 1969.

28. Denny FW, Wannamaker LW, Brink WR, et al: Prevention of rheumatic fever; treatment of preceding streptococcic infection. JAMA 143:151–153, 1950.

29. Devine LF, Johnson DP, Hagerman CR, et al: The effect of minocycline on menin-gococcal nasopharyngeal carrier state in naval personnel. Am J Epidemiol 93:337–345, 1971.

30. DuPont HL, Hornick RB: Clinical approach to infectious diarrheas. Medicine (Baltimore) 52:265–270, 1973.

31. Durack DT, Petersdorf RG, Beeson PB: Penicillin prophylaxis of experimental S. viridans endocarditis. Trans Assoc Am Physicians 85:222–230, 1972.

32. Farid LZ, Bassily S, Lehman JS Jr, et al: A comparative evaluation of the treatment of Schistosoma mansoni with niridazole and potassium antimony tartrate. Trans R Soc Trop Med Hyg 66:119–124, 1972.

33. Ferebee SH: Controlled chemoprophylaxis trials in tuberculosis. A general review. Bibl Tuberc 26:28–106, 1970.

34. Frenkel JK, Weber RW, Lunde MN: Acute toxoplasmosis. Effective treatment with pyrimethamine, sulfadiazine, leucovorin, calcium, and yeast. JAMA 173:1471–1476, 1960.

35. Friedberg CK, Rosen KM, Bienstock PA: Vancomycin therapy for enterococcal and Streptococcus viridans endocarditis. Successful treatment of six patients. Arch Intern Med (Chicago) 122:134–140, 1968.

36. Garnes HA: Doxycycline levels in serum and prostatic tissue in man. Urology 1:205–207, 1973.

37. Genster HG, Andersen MJ: Spinal osteomyelitis complicating urinary tract infection. J Urol 107:109–111, 1972.

38. Glenwright HD, Sidaway DA: The use of metronidazole in the treatment of acute ulcerative gingivitis. Br Dent J 121:174–177, 1966.

39. Golbert TM, Patterson R: Pulmonary allergic aspergillosis. Ann Intern Med 72:395–403, 1970.

40. Gold H: Anthrax, a report of one hundred seventeen cases. Arch Intern Med 96:387–396, 1955.

41. Goodman JS, Koenig MG: Nocardia infections in a general hospital. Ann NY Acad Sci 174:552–567, 1970.

42. Greenough WB, Gordon RS Jr, Rosenberg IS, et al: Tetracycline in the treatment of cholera. Lancet 1:355–357, 1964.
43. Griffin FM Jr: Failure of metronidazole to cure hepatic amebic abscess. N Engl J Med 288:1397, 1973.
44. Guttler RB, Counts GW, Avent CK, et al: Effect of rifampin and minocycline on meningococcal carrier rates. J Infect Dis 24:199–205, 1971.
45. Hardin JW, Braddock G, Croydon EA: Successful treatment of osteomyelitis caused by Pseudomonas aeruginosa. J Clin Pathol 23:653–656, 1970.
46. Harris NH: Some problems in the diagnosis and treatment of acute osteomyelitis. J Bone Joint Surg (Brit) 42B(3):535–541, 1960.
47. Heineman HS, Braude AI: Anaerobic infection of the brain. Observations in eighteen consecutive cases of brain abscess. Am J Med 35:682–697, 1963.
48. Henderson RH, chairman: Venereal Disease Control Advisory Committee, Gonorrhea CDC recommended treatment schedules 1974. 23:341–348, 1974.
49. Hoppes WL, Lerner PI: Nonenterococcal group-D streptococcal endocarditis caused by Streptococcus bovis. Ann Intern Med 815:588–593, 1974.
50. Hume J, Facio G: An analysis of the results of the treatment of yaws with a single injection of procaine penicillin with 2% aluminum monostearate. Bull WHO 15:1057–1085, 1956.
51. Jawetz E: Chemotherapy of chlamydial infections. Adv Pharmacol Chemother 7:253–282, 1969.
52. Jawetz E, Gunnison JB: Determination of sensitivity to penicillin and streptomycin of enterococci and streptococci of viridans group. J Lab Clin Med 35:488–496, 1950.
53. Juel-Jensen B, MacCallum F: Herpes Simplex, Varicella and Zoster: Clinical Manifestations and Treatment. Philadelphia, J.B. Lippincott, 1972.
54. Kahn DS, Pritzker KP: The pathophysiology of bone infection. Clin Orthop 96:12–19, 1973.
55. Kanyuck DO, Welles JS, Emmerson JL, et al: The penetration of cephalosporin antibiotics into bone. Proc Soc Exp Biol Med 136:997–999, 1971.
56. Karl RC, Mertz JJ, Veith FJ, et al: Prophylactic antimicrobial drugs in surgery. N Engl J Med 275:305–308, 1966.
57. Kass EH, Sossen HS: Prevention of infection of urinary tract in presence of indwelling catheters. JAMA 169:1181–1183, 1959.
58. Kaufman HE, Wood RM: Mycotic keratitis. Am J Ophthalmol 59:993–1000, 1965.
59. Kedes LH, Siemienski J, Braude AI: The syndrome of the alcoholic rose gardener. Sporotrichosis of the radial tendon sheath. Report of a case cured with amphotericin B. Ann Intern Med 61:1139–1141, 1964.
60. Kessel JF, Thooris GC, Bambridge B: Use of diethylcarbamazine (hetrazan or notezine) in Tahiti as aid in control of filariasis. Am J Trop Med 2:1050–1061, 1953.
61. Khan W, Ross S, Rodriguez W, et al: Haemophilus influenzae. Type B resistant to ampicillin. JAMA 229:298–301, 1974.
62. Kienitz M: Cephalosporin antibiotics in the treatment of acute osteomyelitis in children. Postgrad Med J 47:Suppl:87–90, 1971.
63. Klein JO, Eickhoff TC, Finland M: Gentamicin: activity in vitro and observations in 26 patients. Am J Med Sci 248:528–544, 1964.
64. Koenig MG, Kaye D: Enterococcal endocarditis. Report of nineteen cases with long-term follow-up data. N Engl J Med 264:257–264, 1961.
65. Kristinsson A, Bentall HH: Medical and surgical treatment of Q-fever endocarditis. Lancet 2:693–697, 1967.
66. Lane SL, Kutscher AH, Chaves R: Oxytetracycline in treatment of orocervical facial actinomycosis; report of seven cases. JAMA 151:986–988, 1953.
67. Leading Article: Prevention of rheumatic fever. Br Med J 1:1625, 1965.
68. Lehr D: Inhibition of drug precipitation in urinary tract by the use of sulfonamide mixtures, sulfathiazole-sulfadiazine mixture. Proc Soc Exp Biol Med 58:11–14, 1945.
69. Lerner PI, Weinstein L: Infective endocarditis in the antibiotic era. N Engl J Med 274:199–206, 1966.
70. Lewis R, Gorback S, Altner P: Spinal Pseudomonas chondroosteomyelitis in heroin users. N Engl J Med 286:1303, 1972.
71. Light RW, Dunham TR: Vertebral osteomyelitis due to Pseudomonas in the occasional heroin user. JAMA 228:1272, 1974.
72. Lopes CF, Alvarenga RJ, Cisalpino EO, et al: Tratamento da cromonicose sela 5-fluorocitosina. Primeiros resultados. Hospital (Rio) 75:1335–1342, 1969 (Por).

73. Lucas AO, Oduntan SO, Gilles HM: Niridazole in guinea worm infection. Ann NY Acad Sci 160:729–739, 1969.
74. Mandell GL, Vest TK: Killing of intraleukocytic *Staphylococcus aureus* by rifampin: in-vitro and in-vivo studies. J Infect Dis 125:486–490, 1972.
75. Martin CM, Bookrajian EN: Bacteriuria prevention after indwelling urinary catheterization; a controlled study. Arch Intern Med (Chicago) 110:703–711, 1962.
76. McCloskey RV, Green MJ, Eller J, et al: Treatment of diphtheria carriers: Benzathine penicillin, erythromycin, and clindamycin. Ann Intern Med 81:788–791, 1974.
77. McVay LV Jr, Sprunt DH: Long-term evaluation of aureomycin in the treatment of actinomycosis. Ann Intern Med 38:955–966, 1953.
78. Miller RP, Bates JH: Pleuropulmonary tularemia. A review of 29 patients. Am Rev Resp Dis 99:31–41, 1969.
79. Modell W: Malaria and victory in Vietnam. The first battle against drug-resistant malignant malaria is described. Science 162:1346–1350, 1968.
80. Moore RA: The cellular mechanism of recovery after treatment with penicillin. I. Subacute bacterial endocarditis. J Lab Clin Med 31:1279–1293, 1946.
81. Perera DR, Western KA, Schultz MG: Niclosamide treatment of cestodiasis: clinical trials in the United States. Am J Trop Med Hyg 19:610–612, 1970.
82. Perine PL, Krause DW, Awoke S, et al: Single-dose doxycycline treatment of louse-borne relapsing fever and epidemic typhus. Lancet 2:742–744, 1974.
83. Perrin JM, Charney E, MacWhinney JB, et al: Sulfisoxazole as chemoprophylaxis for recurrent otitis media; a double-blind crossover study in pediatric practice. N Engl J Med 291:664–667, 1974.
84. Pichler H, Knothe H, Spitzy KH, et al: Treatment of chronic carriers of *Salmonella typhi* and *Salmonella paratyphi* B with trimethoprim-sulfamethoxazole. J Infect Dis 128:Suppl:743–744, 1973.
85. Record CO, Skinner JM, Sleight P, et al: Candida endocarditis treated with 5-fluorocytosine. Br Med J 1:262–264, 1971.
86. Sarosi GA, Parker JD, Doto IL, et al: Chronic pulmonary coccidioidomycosis. N Engl J Med 283:325–329, 1970.
87. Schneider WF, Chapman S, Schulz VB, et al: Prevention of streptococcal pharyngitis among military personnel and their civilian dependents by mass prophylaxis. N Engl J Med 270:1205–1212, 1964.
88. Schroeter AL, Lucas JB, Price EV, et al: Treatment for early syphilis and reactivity of serologic tests. JAMA 221:471–476, 1972.
89. Shronts JS, Rynearson TK, Wolinsky E: Rifampin alone and combined with other drugs in *Mycobacterium kansasii* and *Mycobacterium intracellulare* infections of mice. Am Rev Resp Dis 104:728–741, 1971.
90. Simon HJ, Miller RC: Ampicillin in the treatment of chronic typhoid carriers. Report on fifteen treated cases and a review of the literature. N Engl J Med 274:807–815, 1966.
91. Smith CB, Purcell RH, Chanock RM: Effect of amantadine hydrochloride on parainfluenza type 1 virus infections in adult volunteers. Am Rev Resp Dis 95:689–690, 1967.
92. Smith CB, Wilfert JN, Dans PE, et al: In-vitro activity of carbenicillin and results of treatment of infections due to *Pseudomonas* with carbenicillin singly and in combination with gentamicin. J Infect Dis 122:Suppl:S14–28, 1970.
93. Snyder MJ, Perroni J, Gonzalez O, et al: Trimethoprim-sulfamethoxazole in the treatment of typhoid and paratyphoid fevers. J Infect Dis 128:Suppl:S734–737, 1973.
94. Stamey TA, Meares EM Jr, Winningham DG: Chronic bacterial prostatitis and the diffusion of drugs into prostatic fluid. J Urol 103:187–194, 1970.
95. Tally FP, Sutter VL, Finegold SM: Metronidazole versus anaerobes. In vitro data and initial clinical observations. Calif Med 117:22–26, 1972.
96. Tattersall MH, Spiers AS, Darrell JH: Initial therapy with combination of five antibiotics in febrile patients with leukaemia and neutropenia. Lancet 1:162–165, 1972.
97. Tomeh MO, Starr SE, McGowan JE, et al: Ampicillin-resistant *Haemophilus influenzae* type B infection. JAMA 229:295–297, 1974.
98. Trautman JR: The management of leprosy and its complications. N Engl J Med 273:756–758, 1965.
99. Turck M, Clark RA, Beaty HN, et al: Cefazolin in the treatment of bacterial pneumonia. J Infect Dis 128:Suppl:S382–385, 1973.

99a. Utz JP, Garriques IL, Sande MA, et al: Therapy of cryptococcosis with a combination of flucytosine and amphotericin B. J Infect Dis 132:368–373, 1975.

100. Van Cutsem JM, Thienpont D: Miconazole, a broad-spectrum antimycotic agent with antibacterial activity. Chemotherapy 17:392–404, 1972.

101. Waldvogel FA, Medoff G, Swartz MN: Osteomyelitis: a review of clinical features, therapeutic considerations and unusual aspects. N Engl J Med 282:198–206, 1970.

102. Western KA, Perera DR, Schultz MG: Pentamidine isethionate in the treatment of Pneumocystis carinii pneumonia. Ann Intern Med 73:695–702, 1970.

103. Williams J, Reeves D, Condie A, et al: The Treatment of Bacteriuria in Pregnancy. In Urinary Tract Infection. Edited by O'Grady F and Brumfitt W. New York, Oxford University Press, 1968, pp. 160–169.

104. Wittner M, Tanowitz H: Paromomycin therapy of human cestodiasis with special reference to hymenolepiasis. Am J Trop Med Hyg 20:433–435, 1971.

105. Wolinsky E, Gomez F, Zimpfer F: Sporotrichoid Mycobacterium marinum infection treated with rifampin-ethambutol. Am Rev Resp Dis 105:964–967, 1972.

106. Young LS, Bickness DS, Archer BG, et al: Tularemia epidemia: Vermont, 1968. Forty-seven cases linked to contact with muskrats. N Engl J Med 280:1253–1260, 1969.

107. Young MD, Jeffery GM, Morehouse WG, et al: Comparative efficacy of bephenium hydroxynaphthoate and tetrachloroethylene against hookworm and other parasites of man. Am J Trop Med 9:488–491, 1960.

INDEX

Page numbers in *italics* indicate illustrations. Page numbers followed by (t) indicate tables.

Fluorinated pyrimidines, chemical structure of, 13, *14*
5-Fluorocytosine, absorption of, after oral administration, 68(t)
action of, 32, 35(t)
chemical structure of, 13, *14*
distribution of, in central nervous system, 84
excretion of, during renal failure, 91
minimum inhibitory concentrations effective against fungi, 51(t)
resistance to, 61, *62*
toxic effects of, in blood, 101(t), 103
5-Fluorouracil, chemical structure of, 13, *14*
Food, effect on absorption of antibiotics, 70
Francisella tularensis, drug sensitivity of, 47(t)
infection with, treatment of, 156, 183
Fungal dermal infections, 184–185
Fungemia, treatment of, 180
Fungi, cytoplasmic membrane of, effect of amphotericin B on, 22, *25*
drug resistance in, to 5-fluorocytosine, 61, *62*
drug sensitivity to, 50, 51(t)
mechanisms of drug action in, 25
Fungus infection, of kidney, treatment of, 169
Furunculosis, treatment of, 183
Fusobacterium, drug sensitivity of, 44(t), 46(t), 47(t)
in Vincent's angina, treatment of, 150
Fusobacterium septicemia, metronidazole treatment of, *152*

Gangosa, treatment of, 151
Gastrointestinal tract, toxic effects on, of antimicrobial drugs, 117–118
of clindamycin, 115(t), 118
of lincomycin, 115(t), 118
of neomycin, 115(t), 117–118, *118*, *119*
Genetic exchange, as cause of drug resistance, 57
Genital herpes, treatment of, 167
Genital infections, treatment of, 170
Gentamicin, absorption of, after intramuscular administration, 72(t)
action of, against staphylococci, 43
as cause of deafness, 110
chemical structure of, 7
inactivated by carbenicillin, 139, 139(t), *140*
interaction with ampicillin, 139
sensitivity of gram-negative bacilli to, 47(t)
toxic effects of, in nervous system, 110, 114(t)

Giardiasis, treatment of, 160
Glomerular filtration, of antimicrobial drugs, 75
Gonococcal infections, treatment of, 163, 175, 188–190. See also entries under *Neisseria.*
Gonococcal ophthalmia, prophylaxis for, 195
Gonococcal ophthalmitis, treatment of, 190
Gonococci, drug resistance in, 61
drug sensitivity of, 40, 41(t), 42(t), 43, 52(t)
to cephalosporins, 42(t)
to penicillin, 40, 41(t)
to spectinomycin, 44
to tetracyclines, 42(t)
Gradient plate method, 38, *40*
Gram-negative bacilli, effect of penicillin on, *22*
peptide chains in, 19, *19*
Granuloma inguinale, treatment of, 167
Granulomatous hepatitis, treatment of, 161–162
Griseofulvin, absorption of, after oral administration, 68(t)
action of, against fungi, 51
chemical structure of, 10, *10*
toxic effects of, in skin, 115(t), 121

Half-lives, of antimicrobial drugs, 90(t)
Helminthiasis, treatment of, 160–161
Hematogenous osteomyelitis, treatment of, 192, 193
Hemodialysis, effect on carbenicillin, *93*
effect on kanamycin, *93*
effect on sulfadiazine, 94(t)
Hemolytic anemias, caused by chloramphenicol, 102
Hemophilus aphrophilus infections, treatment of, 172
Hemophilus ducreyi infection, treatment of, 185
Hemophilus influenzae, drug sensitivity of, 44(t), 45, 46(t), 47(t), 48, 52(t), 54
Hemophilus influenzae epiglottitis, treatment of, 149, 152
Hemophilus influenzae infections, treatment of, 155, 157, 171, 174, 188
Hemophilus influenzae meningitis, treatment of, 84, 171, 174
Hepatic excretion, of antimicrobial drugs, 76–79
Hepatic fascioliasis, treatment of, 162
Hepatic infections, treatment of, 161–164
Hepatic insufficiency, effect on antimicrobial drugs, 94–95
effect on carbenicillin, 95
Hepatitis, granulomatous, treatment of, 161–162